DO YOU KNOW . . .

- When a pain in the middle of your belly is a case of indigestion . . . or a life-threatening ulcer

- Why chest pain that's worse when a person is lying down requires immediate medical attention

- What serious infection causes dark spots on the fingernails

- When a momentary "gray curtain" lowering over an eye may be a lifesaving warning sign

- Why a parent should seek expert help if a child has five or more moles

KNOWLEDGE IS POWER.
GET THE ANSWERS YOU NEED IN . . .

YOUR BODY'S RED LIGHT WARNING SIGNALS

Other Books by the Authors

YOUR BODY'S
RED LIGHT
WARNING SIGNALS

•

Medical Tips That Can Save Your Life

*Including a Section on
Lifesaving Pediatric Tips!*

**NEIL SHULMAN, M.D., JACK BIRGE, M.D.,
AND JOON AHN, M.D.**

A DELL BOOK

Published by
Dell Publishing
a division of
Random House, Inc.
1540 Broadway
New York, New York 10036

This book is not intended as a substitute for medical advice of physicians. The reader should regularly consult a physician about matters relating to his or her health and particularly regarding any symptoms that may require diagnosis or medical attention.

ISBN: 0-440-23461-1

Designed by Jeff Ward

Printed in the United States of America

Published simultaneously in Canada

April 1999

10   9   8   7   6   5   4   3   2

OPM

Acknowledgments

Parts Four and Five, on pediatrics, was written by Joy Lawn, M. D. We appreciate her dedication to the health of children.

Christine Zika, our editor, was delightful to work with. She was objective, insightful, and provided invaluable guidance as we worked on this book.

We'd like to thank the hundred of folks in the health profession who reviewed this book with a red pen in hand. Thanks, gang!

Peter Abramson, James Adkins, Helmut Albrecht, J. Richard Amerson, Carol Arnold, Brent Beaird, Justin Bennet, Gregory S. Berns, Christel Biltoft, Allan Bleich, Laurie Boden, Charles Brown, Vickie Brown, James N. Burt, Cassie Cameron, Grant Carlson, Emily Chang, Larry Chang, Emil Chynn, Steve Clements, Leigh Cole, Marius Commodore, Jerard Cranman, Farida DaCosta, Sue Daniel, Bill Davis, Harry Delcher, Donna Dent, Alan Dosik, Arlene Drack, Mike Duffell, Henry Edelhauser, Quinton Foster, Robert Franch, Toyomi Fukushima, Tom Gable, Brenda Garza, Amy Ghiz, Tom Gilmore, Mark Gloger, Russell Gore, Susan Gorman, Charlene Grim, John Gutheil, Dallas Hall, Joe Havlik, Ted Hersh, Joanne Higa, David Holden, Clair Hopkins, Jim Hotz, Celene Howard, Marie Hunter, Bill Hutchinson, Scott Isaacs, Debbie Juncos, Maureen Kelley, Elaine Kennedy, Alison Lauber, Joanna Lawn, Stephen Lawn, Timothy Lawn, Joyce Lee, Erin Lepp, David Levine, Richard and Linda Levinson, Robyn Levy, Fred Lewis, Richard Lewis, Jeffrey Linzer, Scott Lopata, Cindy Ma, Lois Manuel, Luis Marrero, Jonathan Masor, Douglas Mattox, Achintya Maulick, Toni Meador, Melissa Meldrum, Ken Miller, James

Mills, Lori Mills, Stanley Milobsky, Brooks Moore, Mel Moore, Carla Mosby, Ann Motes, Pat Murrah, Jim Neel, Melissa Neiman, Jeff Ng, Wilberto Nieves Neira, Fiona O'Reilly, Gonzalo Orejas, Larry Phillips, Jeffrey Pine, Allan and Susan Platt, Ed Portman, Sue Pressman, Jim Reed, Stanley Riepe, Linda Robinson, Stephen Rockower, Ivor Royston, Grace Rozycki, David B. Rye, Delia Bowman Sattin, Marin Schulman, Ira Schwartz, Richard Seestedt, Purna Sharma, Larry Shulman, Stan Shulman, Bob Shuman, Reeta Sinha, Cynthia Smith, Bob Sobel, Mia J. Sohn, Sid Stein, Henry Storch, Ty Sumner, Todd Stolp, Tim Sullivan, Jean R. Sumner, Joshua Tarkan, Earle Taylor, Jerry Thomas, Naveen Thomas, Thomas Vandergast, Glenna Vitch, Jonathan Waltuck, Fadi Wanna, Eleanor Wood, and Jerry Yuan

and others . . .

Elizabeth Rone, a wonderfully talented artist, made a lot of concepts easier to understand by contributing her artwork.

Many diagrams in this book also come from the book *Let's Play Doctor* (ISBN 0-15-503620-3), available from Rx Humor, 2272 Vistamont Drive, Decatur, GA 30033; tel: (404) 321-0126; fax: (404) 633-9198; Web site: www.dochollywood.com.

Life is a gift.

Practice damage control.

Contents

Appendixes

Introduction

Medical Tips That Can Save Your Life

Most people do not know when to see a doctor. Aches and pains, lumps and bumps—when are these potentially life-threatening? When is it crucial that you get to a doctor within the next few days, hours, or even minutes? Whether you are healthy or ill, there are important medical facts you need to know that can save your life.

Doctors are saddend and frustrated when a patient dies because he or she did not seek medical attention in time. This book has been written as a quick reference guide to use when you or your loved ones have a new pain, a new diagnosis, or a visible bodily change. The goal of this book is to save lives by getting you to a doctor before it is too late.

Whether it is blood in your urine, a stiff neck with a headache and fever, unequal pupils, or red specks in your fingernails, you need to know certain facts about these conditions immediately. The book is designed to highlight urgent warning signs and provide crucial medical tips. It is concise and easy to read, with a few paragraphs about each point.

Routine reference to this book may save your life. Keep it in an easily accessible spot in your home, and get in the habit of checking its pages whenever something unfamiliar happens with your body. Also, refer to it when a friend or relative complains of an ailment. This book is designed to give you a clear, concise statement about potentially life-threatening signs or symptoms. Whenever possible these are listed in order in the Table of Red Light Warning Signals, from head to toe, so you can find them easily.

Owning this book is almost like having an emergency room doctor on your shelf.

How to Use This Book

The First Tier of Health

Keeping healthy involves preventive maintenance as well as the ability to identify diseases early, when treatment is most effective. Taking care of your body is analogous to taking care of your car. The preventive measures for an automobile include oil changes, maintaining fluid levels, and tune-ups. The same goes for your body. Getting adequate exercise, eating a low-fat, high-fiber diet, getting immunized, and sticking to a mentally healthy lifestyle can keep your body humming smoothly. Just as you uncover potential problems with your car by checking your oil and the pressure in your tires, you should have your body checked to detect unsafe levels of blood pressure and cholesterol and early signs of cancer (a routine Pap smear and mammogram, sigmoidoscopic exam, and scan). Many excellent preventive health books address these issues.

The Second Tier of Health

This book addresses the second tier of maintaining your health: identifying your body's red light warning signals. Responsible drivers keep an eye on their car's dashboard lights so that they will be able to address problems immediately. Repairing a leaking radiator or replacing an alternator can prevent the car from dying on the highway. Likewise, your body flashes signals—symptoms and signs—that can warn you of potential problems. If corrected early, you can remain healthy.

When something goes wrong with your car that you cannot identify, the owner's manual is a smart place to turn for information. The challenge of this book is to be an easy-to-access, reader-friendly owner's manual that highlights many of the most common warning signals of your body.

In order to assemble the material in this book, we've mixed our own clinical experience—which adds up to more than 150,000 hours of patient care—with the advice of hundreds of health professionals. **It is not possible to include a reference to every important symptom and sign. Therefore you should always consult your doctor whenever you have a concern.** However, we do hope that this book will help you articulate your problem to your doctor, especially at this time, when the system of health care delivery is imposing so many limitations on your physician's time.

Head to Toe

We have listed, by body part, many of your red light warning signals, starting from your head and going to your toes.

If you have a symptom or find an abnormality on your body, simply look it up in our Table of Red Light Warning Signals by its location on your body. If the problem is not location specific, look in Part Two of the book, which covers warning signs associated with your entire body, such as fever or seizures. Part Three deals with pregnancy and postpregnancy. Although Parts One, Two, and Three list signs and symptoms that can apply to children or teens, Part Four addresses specific pediatric red lights. Also, an alphabetical listing of topics is available in the index at the back of the book.

Most people keep the owner's manual for their car in the glove box or another special place where they can find it easily and quickly. Do the same with this book: Keep it in an easy-to-find location. Though we hope you will not need it, one day it might save your life—or the life of your child, a friend, or family member.

. . . AND KEEP IN MIND

External factors can cause or contribute to an ailment, whether it be toxins in the water from a leaking waste dump, too much exposure to the sun, certain foods, an impure herb, an overdose of vitamins, or starting or stopping a medication. When certain medicines are taken together, they can interact, causing side effects. Learn about the medicines you are taking. Patient package inserts are available from the drugstore. Also, feel comfortable discussing with your doctor and pharmacist the actions, side effects, and interactions of your medicines.

How to Use the Table of Red Light Warning Signals

This book opens with an extensive Table of Red Light Warning Signals, which also serves as a reference guide. Look up your specific symptom or sign and then simply turn to the page or tip number.

Notation: (1) The signs and symptoms listed in this table sometimes occur alone and sometimes in combination. This varies from person to person. (2) It is important to take these red light warning signals seriously, because often effective treatments are available. (3) The tips often refer you to a doctor; however, there are many other excellent members of the health professional team, including nurse practitioners, physician assistants, and midwives, etc., whom you may encounter. (4) The tips may recommend that you seek care at an emergency room. When deciding whether to call an ambulance (911 in most locations in the United States), consider response time as well as your or another person's ability to safely drive to the hospital. Also consider that an ambulance can often provide treatment at the site and can better transport people who are sick. (5) It is impossible for this book to be all inclusive; therefore always seek advice from a doctor if you have a concern about a sign or symptom. The human body's reaction to disease varies and there are always exceptions to the usual presentation of an illness.

For additional tips for children, see PART FOUR.

Table of Red Light Warning Signals

Eyelids
    A Droopy Eyelid, Double Vision, and/or

Vision Abnormalities
  Blurred Vision
    when Pregnant, with Swelling, Upper-Right
      or Middle Belly Pain Under
      the Breastbone,
      Headaches, Dizziness, and/or

  Double Vision
    Alone or with a Droopy Eyelid
      and/or Unequal

Cough

Chest Pain and Chest Discomfort

Irregular Heartbeats and Heart Sounds
Heart Beating Inside Your Head, Usually in

Bowel Movement

Pain

Form and Frequency

Color

Freckles, Moles, Bumps, Warts, Lumps, Plaques, and Patches

PART TWO: General Symptoms and Signs (More Common in Adults): Not Body Part–Specific Conditions

PART THREE: Pregnancy and Postpregnancy

Introduction: Preventive Measures to Increase the
Chances of Delivering a Healthy Baby

PART FOUR: Pediatrics: Body Part–Specific Conditions

(Although more common in adults, Parts One, Two, and
Three all list red light warning signals that can occur in
children.)

Face, Mouth, Throat, and Neck

Arms, Hands, Fingers, and Nails

PART ONE

•

Body Part–Specific Health Problems (More Common in Adults), from Head to Toe

•

Head

Headache

Tip 1:

A sudden, agonizing headache, more severe than any you have felt before, could mean you are bleeding in the brain. This event is an emergency.

Most headaches are caused by tension, stress, sinus infection, allergy, and/or fatigue. They tend to worsen as the day goes on and will go away with an over-the-counter medication or rest. But if you should ever get a sudden, severe headache that you might consider the worst headache of your life, keep in mind that this is the common initial symptom of a potential hemorrhage. The headache often comes on during physical exertion. Again, this event is a medical emergency.

In addition, if a friend or family member complains

of a new severe headache and then becomes sleepy or difficult to awaken, it may also be a hemorrhage in the brain and a medical emergency.

Subarachnoid hemorrhage is a medical term for bleeding around the brain into a compartment known as the subarachnoid space. Your skull, which acts like a tight-fitting helmet that protects your brain, does not allow room for the blood that accumulates during a hemorrhage. This results in increased pressure on your brain.

If the subarachnoid hemorrhage is significant, the blood continues to accumulate in the skull, pushing the soft brain tissue aside. Because the brain has the consistency of a ripe strawberry, this action can result in serious damage.

A subarachnoid hemorrhage usually results from an aneurysm in the brain. Aneurysms (weakened areas on the walls of arteries) may be congenital (that is, you are born with the artery defect) or they may be acquired, such as after a serious injury to the head. They may also be the result of cocaine or amphetamine abuse. The symptoms of hemorrhage in the brain include a severe headache, vomiting, dizziness, seizures, blackouts, sleepiness, slurred speech, double vision, unequal pupil size, and/or mental confusion. Often only the severe headache is present, which sometimes may improve briefly, only to be followed by coma. If you experience "the worst headache of your life," it is advisable to at least contact a doctor immediately.

Early diagnosis is important because one in five people dies from this condition without medication and/or surgery (which includes preventing the bleeding, stopping the bleeding, or removing the blood clot). If a coma follows the headache, the chance of recovery is poor. Fortunately, subarachnoid and other brain hemorrhages are not common.

Tip 2:

Brain tumors usually cause headaches that get progressively worse. These headaches may get especially bad around two A.M. Other signs, such as seizures, weakness, or loss of sensation in a part of the body, can also occur.

One of the main characteristics of a brain tumor is growth. Headaches will worsen as the tumor grows; therefore, if you have been having the same type of headache for more than two years, it is most likely *not* a brain tumor. If your headache seems to be worsening over time, look for other symptoms, such as weakness, visual changes or loss of sensation in a part of the body. Brain tumors usually enlarge to a deadly size within weeks, months, or as long as two years.

The brain sits in clear fluid (spinal fluid) that also surrounds the spinal nerves going down the back from the brain. In a healthy person with a normal sleeping schedule (sleeping at night, awake during the day), spinal fluid pressure is usually highest in the brain and spinal canal around two A.M. Therefore headaches caused by a brain tumor, which increases pressure, will usually get worse around two A.M.

If you experience a headache that becomes progressively worse and/or seizures, or if your headaches are not responding to treatment, you need medical evaluation as soon as possible.

Tip 3:

A headache accompanied by a stiff neck and fever is an indicator of a serious infection called meningitis.

Meningitis is an infection of the lining of the brain (also called the *meninges*) and spinal cord. Outbreaks of meningitis occur all over the world; many result in death. Everyone is at risk of getting meningitis. The disease is not common, but it can be contagious.

Meningitis starts like a flu, with high fever, body aches, an oversensitivity to light, and a severe headache. The telltale sign of meningitis, however, is a stiff neck, except in babies (see Tip 221). If your neck is stiff or if you find you have difficulty touching your chin to your chest, accompanied by fever and a headache, seek medical evaluation. Meningitis must be diagnosed early, because it is a rapidly advancing disease since death can occur as early as thirty-six to forty-eight hours from the onset of symptoms. Any delay in seeking treatment can result in a fatality.

Meningitis is often treatable with antibiotics. If you are exposed to someone diagnosed with meningitis, seek medical advice about preventive measures.

Tip 4:

If you are suffering from symptoms of nausea, headache, and tiredness, think of carbon monoxide poisoning, especially if it happens indoors and to someone else who is living with you.

Poisoning from the inhalation of carbon monoxide continues to cause deaths, despite public awareness of its dangers. Carbon monoxide poisoning can occur very subtly because there is no odor or color to the gas. You do not know the gas is present until illness occurs, and it does not take a lot to make you sick.

Here is a typical scenario: A senior citizen in an older house with a faulty heating system begins to feel bad. The symptoms of carbon monoxide poisoning are weakness, fatigue, nausea, and sometimes chest pain (usually in the elderly). Gums and lips may turn bright red.

The best way to protect yourself against carbon monoxide poisoning is to be aware. Have a heat and air company test the air inside your home for carbon monoxide, and test the heating system for proper exhaust. Do not use kerosene heaters or charcoal grills without proper ventilation. Do not leave your car running in an enclosed area. If any of the symptoms of carbon monoxide poisoning occur while you are in the car, have the exhaust system checked and make sure there are no holes in the floorboard. Inexpensive carbon monoxide monitors are sold at most hardware or department stores that will sound an alarm when levels of carbon monoxide get too high. You can also have your blood tested by a doctor for the presence of carboxyhemoglobin, which will confirm a diagnosis of carbon monoxide poisoning. But note that the levels of carboxyhemoglobin can be altered by exposure to tobacco smoke. Also, the test may be negative if it is performed after you have been away from the carbon monoxide for a period of time.

If you develop any of the red light warning signals of carbon monoxide poisoning, get out of the enclosed area into fresh air immediately. Go to an emergency room for evaluation and treatment.

Tip 5:

If you have tenderness over your temples and/or blurred vision when you have a headache, you may have a serious condition called temporal arteritis.

Temporal arteritis is a relatively rare disease (usually occurring in senior citizens) that causes inflammation of the walls of arteries, especially those of the face and scalp. This condition irritates the walls of the temporal arteries running along the side of your head. These arteries become thickened and inflamed, which may cause headaches and scalp pain, tenderness around the temples, visual disturbances, and sometimes cramping of the jaw muscles while chewing. If the inflammation of the arteries becomes severe enough, blockage of the arteries (stroke) can occur. Blockage of the artery to the eye may result in blurry vision or even vision loss. A stroke can be prevented if diagnosed early and treated. Immediate treatment may prevent complications, while long-term treatment may be necessary to control the ailment. The cause of this disease is unknown.

•
Dizziness

Tip 6:

It is possible for dizziness to suddenly become so severe as to render you nonfunctional and cause you to have a wreck if you are driving a vehicle. Nausea and vomiting may also occur.

Dizziness may mean light-headedness (see Tip 7), or feeling as though you are spinning on a carousel, called vertigo. The balance system consists of multiple factors. To feel balanced, you need to have a normally functioning middle-ear apparatus, and a normal cerebellum (the small area of the brain in the back of the skull responsible for coordination) (see Figure 1). A breakdown in any of these systems can cause you to feel dizzy, which most often occurs with change in body position. Also, a strained neck sometimes causes vertigo.

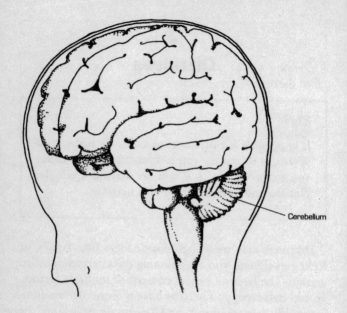

Figure 1. The Brain.

Middle-ear disease can be sporadic, with a sudden, quite severe onset. It can cause vertigo, accompanied by nausea and vomiting. If the attack occurs when you are driving, you could have a serious auto accident.

If you are having vertigo, do not drive, and avoid climbing stairs alone until medical treatment has stabilized the problem. If you experience dizziness with nausea and vomiting, you need medical evaluation as soon as possible.

> **Tip 7:**
>
> Passing out or nearly passing out, with a feeling of dizziness (light-headedness) when you sit up or attempt to stand, is often a result of a drop in blood pressure (orthostatic hypotension). Causes include internal hemorrhage, serious heart irregularities, and severe dehydration. The symptoms can also occur as a side effect of certain medications. The cause may be life-threatening, and injury from a fall due to dizziness may be fatal.

A constant and uninterrupted flow of blood is required by all organs. The brain is the first organ to fail without nutrition and oxygen from the blood. Even a slight change in blood flow to the brain will produce symptoms such as dizziness or fainting.

When you sit up from lying down or when you stand from a sitting position, your blood vessels and heart automatically adjust by narrowing the vessels below the heart and widening the vessels above the heart that supply the brain, assuring adequate blood pressure and blood flow to the brain. If there is not enough blood or fluid in your circulation, from bleeding or dehydration, the automatic adjustments will not provide adequate blood pressure and blood flow to the brain. You will feel dizzy or faint.

It is important to know, however, that heart irregularities can also cause these symptoms. Also, some medications, including water pills (diuretics), certain blood pressure pills, some drugs for psychiatric disorders, and medications for shrinking an enlarged prostate gland, can affect the blood vessels and heart so that they will not adjust properly and prevent the automatic changes from providing adequate blood pressure and blood flow to the brain.

It is important to seek immediate medical evaluation when you begin to get dizzy or faint. If internal hemorrhage, dehydration, or heart irregularities are causing the problem, emergency therapy could save your life. Adjustment in medication that causes these symptoms can sometimes help. The dizziness is particularly dangerous in seniors, who are more subject to serious injuries when they fall.

Tip 8:

Some signs of hypoglycemia (low blood sugar) are weakness, a rapid heartbeat, dizziness, profuse sweating, "acting weird," blackouts, and/or seizures, followed by unconsciousness. Most people who think they have hypoglycemia actually do not, except for diabetics. Although this condition is extremely rare in the general population, it can be fatal if not treated. Drinking fruit juice and putting sugar under the tongue immediately following the onset of symptoms can be lifesaving. Emergency evaluation and treatment are also necessary.

Hypoglycemia means you have a very low blood sugar level (numerically, in the forties or lower). At these levels you become weak, shake, sweat profusely, develop a rapid heart rate, sometimes act "weird," become dizzy, faint (syncopal episode), and/or have seizures followed by unconsciousness. If left untreated, the condition can be fatal.

Hypoglycemia usually occurs when diabetics take too much insulin or too many oral agents for diabetes or do not have adequate input of appropriate foods. A rare cause of very low sugar levels in non-diabetics is a small hormone-producing tumor (insulinoma) in the pancreas, which overproduces insulin. Sudden floods of insulin pass into the bloodstream, causing hypoglycemia, with mental confusion, seizures, and unconsciousness. Occasionally people with hypoglycemia act "weird" and are misdiagnosed as having episodes of mental illness.

Most of these tumors are benign; that is, they are noncancerous. Therefore a complete cure can be obtained by removing the tumor.

Many people think they have hypoglycemia when they actually have minor changes in their circulation or a nervous disorder. They often are misdiagnosed, based on a mild drop in blood sugar, which is insignificant. Although in the general population hypoglycemia is a rare ailment that can be life-threatening, in diabetics it is much more common. Immediate attempts to get sugar into the body by giving fruit juice, putting sugar under the tongue, and/or by giving intravenous sugar water can be lifesaving. Do not attempt to give the victim solid foods. Emergency evaluation and treatment is always necessary.

•

Head Injury

Tip 9:

Head injury: How serious is it?
A head injury that causes nausea, vomiting,
dizziness, drowsiness, mental confusion, or any
loss of consciousness needs immediate medical
evaluation. If any of these symptoms occur hours
or days after a head injury, it constitutes a medical emergency. Always examine the injured person for slurred speech, confusion, unequal pupils,
weakness, or clumsiness in an arm or leg, which
also denote a medical emergency.

Anyone with a head injury of any significance should
be aroused from sleep every hour for the first six hours
(then rechecked every four hours for the next eighteen
hours) after the head injury to make certain they have
not gone into an unconscious state while sleeping. Also,
they should not drink alcoholic beverages or take a sedative or strong pain medication for twenty-four hours.

Note the following three categories of symptoms following a head injury. All are definite warning signs
requiring immediate medical evaluation.

1. Someone who develops symptoms of nausea,
   vomiting, drowsiness, slurred speech, mental confusion, or loss of consciousness even for a short

period of time following a head injury needs immediate medical evaluation and close observation. Any loss of consciousness after a blow to the head indicates a concussion, which is caused by the movement of the brain against the inside of the skull. These symptoms may be a result of anything from mild injury with temporary loss of brain function to a more serious injury with permanent brain damage.

2. **Someone who experiences prolonged unconsciousness after a head injury** has sustained a more serious injury to the brain, which may include hemorrhage into the brain, blood compressing the brain, brain swelling, or spinal cord injury. These are real medical emergencies. The unconscious person needs special treatment until emergency care arrives. Some tips to prevent further damage to the unconscious person are as follows:

a. **Never move the person's head or neck!** Keep the head and neck immobilized until medical personnel arrive. If the person has sustained spinal cord damage, moving the head may worsen the damage or may even be fatal.

In unusual circumstances when someone is vomiting, you may need to gently turn his or her whole body to the side to stop vomitus from getting into the lungs. In this situation the head should be moved only as the shoulders are turned. This maneuver is called a "log roll."

b. **Watch the airway of the unconscious person,** because he or she can develop airway obstruction and even stop breathing. Open the mouth of the injured person and look for food or vomitus that may be blocking the airway. This material may be removed very carefully with your fingers. If the person is still not breathing, administer CPR (see Appendix A).

3. **Someone who appears well shortly after a head injury may still be in danger. He or she may develop symptoms hours later.** When this occurs, failure to obtain emergency treatment can be fatal. Be on the alert for the person who becomes nauseated and vomits, becomes very drowsy, or confused. Unequal pupils and weakness in an arm or leg are important observations, even if the mental status has not changed. These symptoms may indicate complications of the head injury and constitute a true emergency.

These red light warning signals may indicate bleeding in the brain or around the brain, requiring emergency medical intervention. As mentioned earlier, anyone with a head injury of any significance should be aroused from sleep every hour for the first six hours (and every four hours for the next eighteen hours) after the head injury. People over the age of 65 are much more susceptible to serious complications from even a minor head injury.

Tip 10:

If a person becomes loud, abusive, combative, or profane after a head injury, he or she may have a significant brain injury and is in need of emergency medical evaluation.

If you observe someone acting combative or abusive after a head injury, get that person to a doctor as soon as possible, because he or she may have a significant brain injury. A helper who does not realize that this behavior is due to brain injury may think the person is drunk, taking illegal drugs, or just rude. It is very important that combative behavior be recognized as a possible red light warning signal. It may be the only indicator of brain damage that is getting worse.

•

Psychological Problems

Tip 11:

Fatigue, anxiety, and panic disorders may all be related to a medical condition known as depression. In its extreme form, depression can lead to self-destruction. You must know something about it in order to combat it. Effective medicine is available to treat all these disorders.

From the medical perspective, the term *depression* does not necessarily mean feeling "down and withdrawn." The symptoms may be fatigue, loss of appetite, sleeplessness, or headaches. You may have anxiety or a loss of interest in things you normally enjoy. These feelings do not mean that you are "nuts" or a weak person. They may merely mean that you have a chemical imbalance in an area of your brain. They could also be related to excessive alcohol use.

Certain areas of your brain have automatic centers that function without conscious thought to control activities in your body including your heart rate, changes in the size of your pupils or blood vessels, breathing, and sleeping. Normally when you experience an emotional event, these automatic centers create a specific spectrum of symptoms. For example, if someone frightens you, you may feel tightness in your throat, your muscles may become tense, and your heart rate may speed up. Other emotional challenges might trigger one of your automatic brain centers such that you hyperventilate (rapid, deep breathing), have difficulty sleeping, experience headaches and an irritable stomach, and have panic attacks.

If you have a chemical imbalance in one of these automatic centers in your brain, you may experience a variety of these symptoms, even though you have had no emotional experience to trigger them. For example, you may feel fatigued, as though you were exhausted all day, even though you had enough sleep the night before. You may also feel anxious, with the organs of your body reflecting this anxiety, even though nothing has happened to make you anxious. Or you may feel depressed and be withdrawn, even though there appears to be no cause for you to feel this way.

Many effective medications can correct the chemical imbalance in these automatic centers of the brain so that you will not have these symptoms when there is no cause for them. Unfortunately many people do not seek medical treatment because they feel that it is a sign of weakness or that they are just crazy, while in reality they have a chemical imbalance. They may even be suicidal. If you have any of these symptoms and have difficulty controlling them, seek medical evaluation and therapy as soon as possible.

Tip 12:

Delirium means that something is wrong which is affecting the brain, and it could be very serious.

Delirium is usually manifested by an altered state of consciousness, consisting of confusion, distractability, disorientation, and disordered thinking and memory. The person appears detached from his or her surroundings. As this condition progresses, there may be trembling and agitation, even hallucinations and a "complete loss of contact with reality." Many ailments can damage the brain and cause delirium. They include blockage of blood vessels going to the brain, swelling of the brain from high blood pressure, infection of the brain, abnormal chemical levels in the blood, poison, side effects of medication, and lack of oxygen.

When in a state of delirium, a person usually cannot reason, and therefore getting them to medical care may be difficult. He or she may be uncooperative and even combative. But this situation is urgent and requires immediate medical attention. Call for emergency assistance.

Tip 13:

Senility in senior citizens is not always due to Alzheimer's disease or stroke. There is a rare, curable cause that is often associated with an unusual way of walking and/or urinary incontinence.

As they age, senior citizens often develop abnormal personality changes, lose recent memory, and/or become senile. There is a rare cause of these mental changes that can sometimes be cured. Those with the disorder often appear to have difficulty walking or walk in a strange way. The leg muscles are working fine, but the brain does not remember how to use them. One does not have the ability to purposefully initiate a specific movement. In other words the individual may not be able to remember how to walk. When he or she does walk, the pattern of walking seems quite awkward. The condition is often accompanied by urinary incontinence (inability to control the bladder).

The medical name of the condition causing these red light warning signals is *normal pressure hydrocephalus*. It can result from a head injury, brain hemorrhage, or meningitis (an infection in the sac that surrounds the brain). It can also occur without any known cause. It usually appears in senior citizens, but it can occur in younger people.

The brain sits in a clear liquid that flows into the inner chambers of the brain. If something blocks the natural flow of this liquid, too much fluid may accumulate in these chambers. The pressure from the excess fluid damages areas of the brain, causing the symptoms.

The diagnosis can be made with special studies of the brain, including a CT scan or an MRI. If the chambers of the brain are enlarged, normal pressure hydrocephalus may be present.

This rare condition can sometimes be reversed with surgery. One end of a small tube is placed in an inner chamber in the brain. The tube is sewn in place down the neck through the body to the belly cavity, where the excess fluid can flow.

Family members of persons who are senile should discuss the possibility of this diagnosis (normal pressure hydrocephalus) and the pros and cons of medical testing for this ailment with a neurologist (brain specialist).

Also, the discussion should include evaluation of other potentially reversible causes of senility, including decreased thyroid function (hypothyroidism), increased parathyroid function (hyperparathyroidism), vitamin B_{12} deficiency, and side effects of medication.

Tip 14:

A sudden change in personality may not be the result of a primary psychiatric disorder but may occur from chemical changes in the blood or a side effect of certain medications. Personality changes can also be caused by tumors, a brain injury (that may be unwitnessed), and bleeding in the brain.

A sudden change in personality—including anxiety, apathy, confusion, or even psychosis—may be one of the body's red light warning signals of a treatable chemical or physical abnormality in the body including the brain. It is important to seek medical evaluation in order to treat the underlying illness. In many cases medical treatment can reverse the personality disorder.

• Eyes

Eyelids

Tip 15:

If one of your eyelids droops, you're seeing double, and/or your pupils are unequal in size, you may have a ballooning blood vessel (aneurysm) in your brain that could burst, or a brain tumor.

An eyelid that does not move normally, pupils that are unequal in size, and/or seeing double may indicate that the nerve controlling these functions is not transmitting impulses normally (see Figure 2). Any abnormality, in the brain or surrounding structures, that puts pressure on this nerve can cause these signs. A blood vessel that is ballooning out (aneurysm) at a specific location could press on this nerve. These signs may be an early red light warning signal for emergency medical evaluation and brain surgery to contain the blood vessel before it bursts.

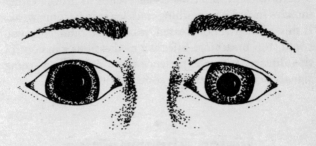

Figure 2. Eyes with Uneven Pupils.

Tip 16:

If your eyelids droop part of the time and you have double vision, or your jaw gets tired while chewing, you may have a serious neurological problem.

Do people ask, "Why don't you open your eyes all the way? You look like you're sleepy." Do your jaws get so tired at times when you are eating that you cannot take another bite? If you have droopy eyelids, weary jaws, difficulty swallowing or general weakness, you may have a potentially serious nerve disorder called myasthenia gravis.

With myasthenia gravis there is a blockage of a

chemical necessary for sending messages through your nerves to certain muscles in your body. Only a weakened nerve signal gets to the muscle. Weakened muscles make it hard to chew and cause your eyelids to droop. Other muscles including breathing muscles may become weak. If this ailment is not treated, it could be fatal since you could stop breathing. Effective medications can control this disease. If you experience these red light warning signals, see your doctor as soon as possible.

•

Vision Abnormalities

Tip 17:

When the view you see becomes narrowed, it may be an important symptom of a pituitary gland tumor, a brain tumor, a stroke, an injury to the retina of the eye, or advanced glaucoma.

When you look straight ahead, usually you can see objects on your right and left side. These are your peripheral visual fields. The loss of a portion of your peripheral visual field is a red light warning signal. This loss causes your vision to be similar to that of a horse wearing blinders.

A simple test to detect this abnormality is to put your right hand over your right eye and put your left hand behind your left ear. While looking straight ahead, move your left hand slowly so that it is reaching out in front of your face. You should be able to detect this movement out of the corner of your left eye even though you are looking straight ahead. Do the same while looking through your right eye. If neither eye picks up your normal peripheral vision, you may have a visual field defect.

Causes of this syndrome include a stroke due to blockage of a blood vessel in the brain, an injury to the retina of the eye, glaucoma, bleeding in the brain, or a tumor in the area of the brain responsible for vision. A tumor of the pituitary gland, located on the underside of the brain, can also cause these symptoms. If the tumor gets large enough, it can press on the nerves from the eyes and cause the visual field loss. Also, the tumor can produce high levels of hormones that may cause a milky white discharge from the nipples and stop or alter menstrual periods. The growth can be controlled medically or surgically.

If you experience a sudden narrowing of vision, you should go to an emergency room. In all cases, you need evaluation by an ophthalmologist.

Tip 18:

If it seems as though a dark gray curtain or haze is going down over one eye or part of your vision and then back up, it can be a sign that you are about to have a stroke.

If it seems as though your vision is clouded by a descending gray curtain—or a blur, haze, mist, or fog— usually for about one to five minutes, it could mean several things. One of the blood vessels leading from your heart into your neck or some of those supplying your brain could be partially blocked. When this happens, the blood vessel to the nerve to the eye *or* the part of the brain responsible for vision is not getting enough blood.

You need to be taken to an emergency room immediately. Emergency treatment may prevent a stroke. If your sight does not return and you see an ophthalmologist (eye doctor) within ninety minutes, he or she may be able to treat you and save your vision.

•

Vision Loss

Tip 19:

A sudden loss of vision in one eye or part of your vision that usually lasts for a few seconds to a few minutes may be the warning sign of a major stroke.

People with this condtion are at high risk of having a major stroke. If you suddenly lose part of your vision for a short period of time, this is a red light warning signal that you need urgent evaluation by your doctor. Sudden eyesight loss is a sign of a blocked blood vessel supplying a nerve to an eye or part of the brain responsible for sight. Emergency treatment to prevent a stroke is necessary. Often a blood thinner is given or surgery is instituted to clean out a blocked artery.

If total vision does not return and you see an ophthalmologist (eye doctor) within ninety minutes, he or she may be able to treat you and save your sight.

•

Ear, Nose, Mouth, Throat, and Neck

Ear

> **Tip 20:**
>
> Gradual hearing loss in one ear sometimes with a sense that the room is spinning around and/or ringing in the ear may be an indication of a tumor of or near the nerve responsible for hearing.
>
> Sudden vertigo and ringing in the ears followed by hearing loss can signal a rare, life-threatening total body disease, which, if treated within two weeks, is potentially curable (Logan's syndrome).

Hearing loss due to aging is a common, gradual process, and many times it is hardly noticed until someone else points it out. Another common source of hearing loss—noise exposure—is also gradual and occurs in both ears. In addition hearing loss is often inherited.

But what about the gradual hearing loss in one ear that may be accompanied by a feeling that the room is spinning around and/or a ringing in the ear? A rare but serious illness that can cause this is a tumor of or near the hearing nerve. Urgent medical evaluation is indicated. Other more common causes of hearing loss and this type of dizziness include an inflammation of the hearing apparatus in the ear. Often no cause can be found, although there may be effective treatments.

Tip 21:

Hearing the sound of your heart beating inside your head usually in association with episodic headaches could mean that you have a blood vessel malformation that can cause a stroke.

It is common to hear your heart beat in your ear when you lie down and place your ear against a pillow. But if you note the onset of pulsating noise similar to a beating heart on one side of your head, and if it is constantly present no matter what your body position, it is abnormal. It could indicate a problem with your ear. It could also be an indication of a blood vessel abnormality inside your head or neck, especially if in association with episodic throbbing headaches on one side of your head.

Veins carry blood to the heart, while arteries carry blood away from the heart. The rare type of blood vessel abnormality most likely to produce these heart-beating sounds is called a dural arteriovenous malformation. This abnormality, often present at birth, is caused by a direct connection of an artery to a vein that significantly increases blood pressure in the veins. As time passes, these malformations may get bigger and begin producing the heartbeat sound with such intensity that it can be heard in the ear closest to the malformation. If you hear the sound of your heart beating in your head, especially with episodic headaches, seek medical evaluation by an ear specialist (otolaryngologist). A blood vessel malformation may need to be repaired so it will not rupture and cause a brain hemorrhage. A more common cause of these symptoms is rapid flow of blood in veins around the ear, which also needs evaluation, but is not as serious.

•

Nose

Tip 22:

Nosebleeds are usually easily controlled but can be fatal in rare cases.

It is possible, though improbable, to bleed to death from a nosebleed. Nosebleeds are especially dangerous if you are taking a blood thinner such as Coumadin. The majority of nosebleeds originate from just inside the nostril on the wall that separates the nostrils, called the septum. Lightly packing the nose with gauze or cotton (with material protruding from the nostrils), sometimes soaked in Afrin or Neosynephrine, can usually control this bleeding. (Make certain there are no contraindications for you to use these medicines by checking the patient package insert.) In addition, external compression such as pinching the soft part of the nose for a full five minutes with the head bent forward and applying an ice pack can help stop the bleeding. These steps will control the majority of nosebleeds. Do not blow your nose for at least six hours after treatment! If you still have a nosebleed after you've tried all these methods, seek medical attention immediately.

Some bleeding sites, deep in the catacombs of the nasal passage, are difficult to access and control. When injured, the major blood vessels located there are more susceptible to severe bleeding. Typically the blood will stream to the back of your throat, requiring constant swallowing. This problem poses a challenge even to the ear-nose-throat specialist. Seek medical help immediately before you lose too much blood.

Nosebleeds are more severe in people with high blood pressure. Most result from a crack or ulcer on the nasal passage, often from dry air, chronic allergic congestion, or a growth called a polyp. If you have a disease or take a drug that impairs blood clotting, including aspirin, or if you routinely drink too much alcohol, you are at particular risk of severe blood loss from a nosebleed.

Tip 23:

Infections of the upper lip or nose can be dangerous and spread to the inside of the head.

You have heard of the Bermuda Triangle and its dangers, but you may not have heard of the "dangerous triangle." The body has one, and it has perils as well. The apex or tip of the triangle is at the forehead between the eyebrows. The angles of the triangle are at the corners of the mouth.

This triangle differs from other areas of the face and head in one very important way: Blood brought to this area by arteries will return to the heart through veins that travel inside the skull rather than through vessels that remain outside the skull.

Why is this important? Germs, which have gained entrance to the circulation in this location, have a direct route to the brain and other structures inside the skull. Infections in the brain can quickly spread to vital centers responsible for normal life functions, and therefore they can be fatal.

An infected bump or boil, or any infection on the upper lip, or inside or outside the nose, holds a greater threat of serious complications than many infections elsewhere on the face or head. Signs of infection are tenderness, warmth, swelling, and redness. When they occur, see your doctor as soon as possible. Due to the seriousness of infection in this locale, you should not delay seeking treatment by using home remedies, except for the most mild surface sores. Picking or squeezing the infected area can spread the infection.

•

Mouth

Tip 24:

Fruity-smelling breath may indicate a serious blood sugar problem when diabetes gets out of control and your blood becomes dangerously acidic.

Diabetes is a condition that results when sugar in your blood is abnormally high, usually because of low levels of insulin, a hormone that is produced in the pancreas. The earliest signs of diabetes include frequent urination and unquenchable thirst. Insulin drives sugar from the blood into cells in your body so they can get nourishment. Diabetes can also be caused by the body not responding to insulin. In untreated diabetes the body no longer burns sugar as its normal source of energy; rather, it burns fat. When fat is burned, it produces acid compounds as by-products, causing the blood to become acidic. Some of the acid is eliminated through the lungs, producing a characteristic fruity-smelling breath. When the acid by-products build up and the blood sugar rises, you may experience extreme thirst, shortness of breath, and/or abdominal pain. Without treatment, coma and death may follow.

The person with diabetes rarely detects the strange-smelling breath odor, so it is important that he or she be informed when this appears. He or she needs emergency medical evaluation. Most people have not smelled this odor before, but it is readily identified as an unusual smell. Unfortunately the smell is sometimes mistaken for alcohol, and the person is misdiagnosed as being drunk because acid in the blood can also make one act in a drunken manner.

Tip 25:

A metallic taste on the tongue or a garlic odor on the breath may indicate arsenic poisoning.

Early signs of arsenic poisoning can be a garlic odor on the breath and a metallic taste on the tongue. Later symptoms of arsenic poisoning are vomiting and a burning, upset stomach. You may also experience tingling and burning in your arms and legs as well as other problems from damage to your nerves. Certain medications (like Biaxin), however, can also give you an abnormal taste.

Arsenic poisoning has been known to occur in incidents of mail-order poisoning. No doubt you've also heard of food supplements or medications being intentionally laced with arsenic and distributed. An early sign of poisoning may be a metallic taste. Call your local poison control center for additional information and advice on appropriate evaluation and treatment.

Tip 26:

A sore inside the mouth, on the tongue, or in the throat that does not heal may be cancer. White spots in these areas may also be a sign of early cancer.

A sore inside the mouth, on the tongue, or in the throat that does not heal within three weeks is considered to be cancer until proven otherwise. A white spot (called leukoplakia), which can be found in the same locations, is potentially precancerous. An ear-nose-throat specialist or a dental surgeon is the best specialist to evaluate this problem. Make an appointment as soon as possible.

Leukoplakia, caused by irritants in the mouth, can be

the result of abrasive contact of the mouth's lining with the rough edge of a tooth or denture, but more commonly it occurs from the use of tobacco. Pouching snuff in the mouth and chewing tobacco are very irritating to surface cells in the mouth, which react and lead to the formation of leukoplakia. If this overgrowth continues, it can evolve into cancer, which can spread to other parts of the body.

Another cause of white spots in the mouth is yeast infections. Yeast infections in the mouths of babies are common because they have a youthful immune system. Yeast infections occur in the mouths of some adults taking antibiotics or steroids. They can also appear as a result of an abnormally weak immune system caused by diseases such as AIDS. If it continues, this symptom warrants a visit to the doctor.

Tip 27:

Any ulcer (sore with superficial loss of tissue) in the mouth that lasts for more than three weeks should be evaluated by your doctor or dentist, an oral surgeon, or an ear-nose-throat specialist to rule out cancer.

Tip 28:

A blue or black spot in the mouth may be a sign of cancer.

Early signs of cancer can appear as a blue or black spot in the mouth. There are other more common causes as well, including stains from silver fillings and normal pigmentation. A dentist or doctor, oral surgeon, or ear-nose-throat physician can determine the cause of the discoloration.

•

Throat

Tip 29:

Epiglottitis can block your airway. If you are gasping with a "seal-like" noise, often associated with a severe sore throat, you need to be seen by a doctor on an emergency basis!

Epiglottitis is an infection of the epiglottis (the flap over the windpipe that stops food from getting into the lungs when you swallow). When infected, the epiglottis swells, blocking the airway.

Epiglottitis is often associated with a severe sore throat, which may be followed by gasping with a "seal-like" sound.

An important warning sign of a potential life-threatening case of epiglottitis is the presence of depressed areas at the neck base, just above the breast-bone, and in the spaces between the ribs. If these areas are noticeably sucked in when you inhale, negative pressure in the chest cavity is potentially being created by a significant blockage of the airway.

If you are experiencing noisy breathing or are struggling to inhale, you may be having difficulty getting air in the lungs. Call for an ambulance (911 in many locations). You need emergency care. (See Tip 199 for information on epiglottitis in babies and children.)

Tip 30:

Persistent hoarseness for more than three weeks may be caused by cancer of the vocal cords or other serious illnesses. Seek medical evaluation by an ear, nose, and throat specialist (otolaryngologist) as soon as possible.

Your voice is generated by the vibrations of your vocal cords, which are located in the area of the throat called the larynx (a structure in the upper part of the breathing tube). Changes in vocal cords can cause hoarseness. Think of it like a guitar string—the thicker the string, the lower the pitch. The more swollen the vocal cord, the lower the pitch, until it becomes a whisper.

The most common causes of hoarseness are irritation of the vocal cords from infection and swelling of the vocal cords from excessive voice use. These conditions usually go away after a few days. Allergies can also contribute to hoarseness; thus the pattern of hoarseness may come and go with the seasons.

Persistent hoarseness (lasting more than three weeks) may be a tip-off to throat cancer, which causes thickening of a vocal cord that does not go away. This occurs more commonly in smokers and in people with reflux of acid from the stomach. A cure is possible with early diagnosis and treatment. Hoarseness can also result from fluid entering the lung when liquids you drink go up your nose when you swallow. This condition may be indicative of a nerve or muscle disorder, or a stroke, or a tumor.

Tip 31:

If food or drink will not go down when you swallow, you may have a partial esophagus obstruction that may lead to or be a sign of cancer.

Difficulty swallowing is a common problem. Most of the time it occurs when eating bulky foods like meat or corn bread. You swallow, and it sticks at a narrowed site of the esophagus (the swallowing tube from mouth to stomach) before finally going down. You feel the food getting stuck in a region underneath the lower area of the breastbone.

Narrowing of the esophagus most often occurs in the lower esophagus. It is often the result of a ring of scar tissue that has formed due to stomach acid refluxing (backing up) into the lower esophagus, irritating and scarring it. As the scarring increases, the constriction or narrowing of the esophagus increases, and more foods get stuck when you swallow. It can progress to the point of complete blockage; relieving the obstruction will require emergency treatment.

A major reason to evaluate this problem early, long before complete blockage occurs, is to prevent the development of cancer of the esophagus, which can arise from a longstanding irritation of the esophagus. A gastroenterologist (doctor expert in the stomach and colon) can insert a special tube with a small video camera into your mouth and down the esophagus. By obtaining a small piece of the esophagus (biopsy), he or she can make a diagnosis to determine whether a longstanding irritation or cancer is present.

Tip 32:

A severe sore throat may be an indication of a throat infection that can close off your airway.

Did you know that a sore throat can close off your airway and cause you to strangle? Three major kinds of infection can endanger the airway: a pus pocket around the tonsils (peritonsillar abscess); an infection in the floor of the mouth, spreading throughout the jaw and around the teeth (Ludwig's angina); and an infection of the epiglottis (the flap over your windpipe that keeps food from entering). You can prevent these infections by seeking treatment for a sore throat before it worsens.

Since sore throats are so common, how will you know when you may be in danger? Usually you get a sore throat, and in a few days you are well. Sometimes you receive antibiotics from a doctor, and your sore throat improves. But occasionally the germs dig deeper into the tissues of the throat and set up an abscess (pus pocket) that can bulge into your airway, narrowing it. Usually the pain will become worse and the fever higher, which means you need further medical treatment.

If you get a sore throat, make sure it gets better over a

forty-eight-hour period. Never let it go longer before seeking medical attention. Be aware that a sore throat after a dental procedure is dangerous since it can spread faster. If you experience hardness or swelling in the floor of your mouth and around the base of your tongue, if you have difficulty opening your mouth, or if you notice drooling of saliva from your mouth, it is an emergency. These more serious throat infections are often much worse on one side of your throat. When you open your mouth and look in the mirror, if the dangling thing hanging in the back of your throat (uvula) does not point down but shifts to one side, go to your doctor or to the emergency room.

Occasionally a sore throat that does not respond to treatment after a number of weeks is caused by a tumor located deep in the throat. These tumors can be seen only when the doctor uses a special small mirror to look in your mouth.

Tip 33:

If you have a severe sore throat with fever and a fiery red rash all over your body, seek medical evaluation right away. You may have scarlet fever. Also, your tongue may look like an intensely red strawberry, and your throat may be red with white splotches.

Scarlet fever is caused by a rare type of the same germ that gives you a strep throat. The germ releases a toxic substance into the bloodstream, which causes a red rash, as well as heart and kidney disease. Your skin may peel off as though you have been sunburned.

Antibiotic therapy is needed as soon as possible to avoid these life-threatening complications.

Tip 34:

If you have a sore throat, followed by fever and joint swelling about two weeks later, watch out. You can get rheumatic fever from strep throat if it is not adequately treated.

Rheumatic fever is a complication of strep throat. It usually occurs two to three weeks after having strep throat. It can cause the joints in your body to become swollen and painful. Fever and swelling are reactions of the body to infection by the germ streptococcus. Rheumatic fever can also affect the heart, causing the heart muscle to become inflamed. It can permanently damage the heart valves.

Rheumatic fever is most common in children over four years old, but it can also occur in adults. Adequate treatment of the initial sore throat is the secret to the prevention of rheumatic fever. If your doctor prescribes a course of antibiotics, make sure you take all of the medicine.

Other complications of a strep infection are acute glomerulonephritis (inflammation of the kidneys) and scarletina (scarlet fever—see Tip 33), the appearance of a scarlet rash (a generalized red rash).

•

Neck

Tip 35:

A lump found in the thyroid gland, at the front base of the neck (under the "Adam's apple" in men), may be cancerous.

The thyroid gland is located in the front base of the neck. If you detect an enlargement or lump in your thyroid gland, make an appointment with your doctor as soon as possible for testing and treatment. Goiter means that your thyroid gland is larger than normal. The three basic kinds of enlargement are:

- A general enlargement of the entire gland, often caused by a disorder of the immune system. It can also be caused by a deficiency of iodine (which is rare).
- A lumpy enlargement of the entire gland, which is usually harmless; occasionally cancer is found in part of the gland.
- A single lump in the gland, which may be cancerous. Thyroid cancer can often be cured with treatment.

Tip 36:

A lump anywhere in the neck can be a sign of a serious illness.

The most serious neck lumps are not associated with thyroid disease (in the front base of the neck). These other lumps are often new, and are found only on one side of your neck. These lumps are often indicative of a lymph node that has been enlarged because of an infection. If the lump is located in the front of your neck, it probably resulted from a throat infection. If the lump is in the back of the neck, it is usually the result of a scalp or ear infection.

These enlarged lymph nodes are often less than an inch thick, and they shrink within fourteen days after the infection has been treated. They have a rubbery, semisoft feel and are tender to the touch.

Lumps in the neck that are present longer than fourteen days, are over one inch in size, are firm or hard in texture, and/or are not tender are more suspicious of cancer of the lymph nodes or cancer that has spread from another site.

These are the general guidelines for examining lymph nodes, but there are exceptions. Seek advice from your doctor if any such lump persists.

•

Arms and Hands

Armpits

Tip 37:

A lump in the armpit may be an enlarged lymph node, indicating a serious illness.

Lumps in the armpit are common. Most are tender sweat glands that have been clogged with deodorants, especially those containing "drying agents." If these glands get infected, they may form large pus pockets and require drainage. Usually lumps from clogged sweat glands can be distinguished from other lumps because you cannot move them separately from the skin with your fingers. A lump that is deep under the skin is usually a lymph node, and when feeling it, you can move the skin separately from the lump.

Enlarged lymph nodes in the armpit are often due to infections in the arm or hand. The most serious cause of an enlarged lymph node is cancer that has spread to that node.

Early medical evaluation of the cause of a lump in the armpit is important, especially because it could be a red light warning signal of treatable cancer. For example, the lump may indicate breast cancer.

•

Arms

Tip 38:

Paralysis, weakness, tingling, burning pains, numbness, confusion, slurred speech, etc., are signs of a stroke, and you should get to an appropriate emergency center immediately. Early treatment may prevent permanent damage to the brain or even save your life.

A stroke may be caused by a blood clot that has formed in one of the arteries that supplies the brain with oxygen (see Figure 3). A stroke can also be caused by a blood clot that has formed in a vessel somewhere else in the body including the heart and has traveled through the blood to a vessel in the brain. The area supplied by the blocked blood vessel is rapidly damaged. The loss of oxygen affects the brain first before any other body organ. A few minutes of oxygen deprivation can result in permanent loss of function.

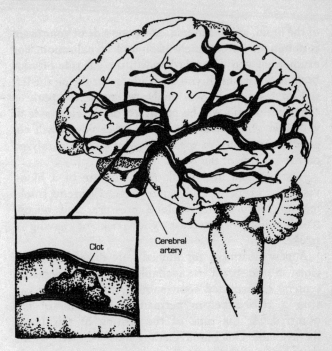

Figure 3. Blood Clot in Brain.

Symptoms of a stroke are related to the particular area of the brain that is involved. If a large vessel is blocked, such as the middle cerebral artery, a large area of the brain will be affected, causing paralysis of one side of the body. If a smaller blood vessel is blocked, then paralysis may be limited to an arm or leg.

The right side of the body is controlled by the left side

of the brain, and vice versa. Also, one side of your brain is dominant for comprehension and verbalization. For example, if you are right-handed, the left side of your brain is dominant. If you have a large stroke on the left side of your brain, you might be unable to speak or comprehend and will be paralyzed on the right side of your body. If the stroke is on the other side, it will not affect your ability to speak, but you will be paralyzed on the left side of the body.

A stroke can also result from rupture of a blood vessel in the brain and hemorrhage. Cigarette smoking, uncontrolled high blood pressure, and uncontrolled diabetes increase your risk of having a stroke.

A new treatment for immediately dissolving blood clots in the brain is available at most emergency centers. If instituted soon enough, the treatment can stop a stroke before permanent brain injury has occurred. At the time of the writing of this book, the available clot buster therapy must be given within three hours of the onset of symptoms in order to work. The sooner the better. Newer medications being developed may work for a longer period of time after symptoms first appear. However, this therapy is not appropriate for all stroke victims. For example, if the stroke is the result of a hemorrhage in the brain, you definitely do not want to get clot buster therapy or a blood thinner.

You need to be aware of stroke symptoms, call for an ambulance and get immediate transportation to an appropriate emergency room. All stroke victims need urgent evaluation even if you are not able to get to medical care in the first three hours. Do not wait!

Tip 39:

A short episode of numbness on one side of your face, slurred speech, weakness in the leg or arm, double vision and/or "vertigo" (an unbalanced feeling), etc., which lasts for only a short period of time (ten minutes to one hour), indicates that a certain area of the brain is not getting enough blood. This is called a TIA (transient ischemic attack).

A TIA is a red light warning signal of a stroke. When a blood clot loose in the circulation gets stuck in a narrow blood vessel going to the brain, it will restrict blood flow and cause abnormal functioning in the area of the brain that is not getting adequate oxygen and nourishment. For example, it could create numbness of the face, slurring of the speech, or weakness of the hands. When the blood clot dissolves on its own, blood flow returns and the symptoms go away. Intermittent rhythm abnormalities of the heart can also cause decreased blood flow to the brain, resulting in these symptoms.

Persons with these red light warning signals require emergency evaluation and therapy because if the next clot is larger or the following heart rhythm abnormality lasts too long, the affected brain tissue may be further damaged and a stroke may occur. Also, once a TIA has occurred it is more likely to recur unless treatment is instituted. If these symptoms develop, do not wait to see if they resolve. Seek immediate emergency care.

•

Hands

> **Tip 40:**
>
> Shaking hands or hand tremors may be the first signs of serious illness, including an overactive thyroid or Parkinson's disease.

Trembling hands may be an early sign of an overactive thyroid. It is important to diagnose this disease as early as possible; it can injure the heart. The tremor of an overactive thyroid is usually very fine and hard to see, but it can be made evident by a simple test: Extend your arms with the palms of your hands up, and place a sheet of paper on one of the hands. Shaking of the hand becomes quite evident. Other symptoms of an overactive thyroid are intolerance to heat, sweating, and weakness.

Shaking hands are called hand tremors. You can also have tremors of the head, arms and legs together, or they can be localized to only the head or one arm or leg. They may be fine and barely noticeable, or they may be coarse and shake the coffee out of a cup. They may also get worse with attempts at coordinated movements such as touching the tip of your nose with your index finger (that is, the closer your finger gets to your nose, the worse the tremor gets). Also, it is more apparent when you try to sign your name. Most of these tremors are probably inherited but appear later in life.

Parkinson's disease also causes a tremor as well as muscle rigidity, which is much more disabling because it impedes movement. The tremor is expressed as though you are rolling a pill between your fingers at rest. It is accompanied by an expressionless face and stooping shoulders with a shuffling walk. Parkinson's disease is a brain disorder in which excessive nerve impulses flow from the brain. In senior citizens Parkinson's-like disorders are usually caused by multiple small strokes.

The most common cause of tremors in the young is substance abuse. But you do not have to be an alcoholic or on crack cocaine to develop tremors. Often the scenario involves a busy young executive under stress, working long hours, drinking too much coffee, then drinking three or four Scotch and sodas every night to "wind down," and/or heavily smoking. This person begins to notice shaking hands in the mornings. The shaking signals the beginning of dependency on the substance, and it first appears when one stops the drinking or smoking. It is a toxic effect on the central nervous system. Often it gets worse if the person does not stop drinking or smoking.

Certain prescription drugs can also cause tremors. Strong tranquilizers cause them so often that additional medicines may be necessary to prevent the tremors. A relatively new medication for certain stomach disorders (Reglan/metocloprimide) can cause tremors, even a full-blown Parkinson's-like disorder. It clears very slowly when the medication is stopped.

It is important to seek medical evaluation early to determine the cause of your tremor, since treatment may prevent serious additional complications from the underlying problem.

> **Tip 41:**
>
> Smokers sometimes develop slow-healing sores on their fingertips, around their fingernails, or on their toes. These sores may indicate that a serious disease is blocking their arteries.

If you smoke and have sores on your fingertips or toes, you need to stop. These sores are often painful, may occur in one digit only, intermittently blanch white, and are intolerant to exposure to cold. The disease causing this red light warning signal is thromboangiitis obliterans (Buerger's disease).

This ailment causes the inner linings of small to medium-sized arteries to thicken and scar. The blood vessels narrow, impairing circulation and causing damage to the fingers and toes. The damage can be so severe that it leads to gangrene and may ultimately require amputation of the arm and/or leg. Dangerous blood clots can also form in these blood vessels, which potentially can lead to fatal complications. If you notice these changes in your fingers or toes, seek medical advice as soon as possible, and stop smoking.

•

Fingers

> **Tip 42:**
>
> Enlargement of the fingertips widens and deforms the nails and gives them a club-like appearance. It can be an important sign of a serious disease.

Enlargement of the ends of the fingers in club-like fashion occurs insidiously and without pain; therefore it attracts little attention or concern. Ultimately it can result in bone deformity. These changes are commonly seen in inherited heart diseases that impair oxygenation of the blood. It is thought that diseases of the lung, liver, and bowel, including cancer, can also result in these deformities. So if club fingertips appear, make an appointment with your doctor as soon as possible and find out why.

•

Fingernails

> **Tip 43:**
>
> Splinter-like reddish dark spots in the fingernails may be a sign of a serious infection in the heart.

Usually dark spots in the fingernails are due to a prior injury. But splinter hemorrhages in the nails may be due to fragments of infected material breaking off from an infected heart valve and then traveling to the tiny vessels in the fingernail beds under the nails. As the tiny vessels become clogged, the damaged walls begin to leak blood into the surrounding tissue, forming the splinter-like reddish dark spot. Since these hemorrhages are not painful, they may go unnoticed.

A heart valve infection (bacterial endocarditis) is a serious medical condition with a high mortality rate. It usually occurs in individuals who have a heart valve abnormality. Germs that gain entrance to the bloodstream are able to invade a diseased heart valve, multiply, and build a substance called vegetation. Fragments of these vegetations, which are full of germs, can break off and spread throughout the body via the blood. Germs commonly gain entrance into the bloodstream from ordinary dental work. This is why, prior to dental procedures, dentists prescribe antibiotics to patients with heart valve disease. Antibiotics should be given to these patients prior to any medical procedure (with instruments), such as an examination of the colon or bladder.

The use of unclean needles can cause infection of normal heart valves because of the large number of germs it introduces into the bloodstream. This condition is often seen among intravenous drug abusers.

Initially, symptoms of bacterial endocarditis may be insidious such as slight weakness, weight loss, intermittently high fevers and/or chills, tiredness, or joint pains. An infection in a heart valve should be treated on an emergency basis in order to kill the germs before they cause serious damage to the heart.

Tip 44:

Fungus of the nails is often merely unsightly, but certain medicines used in their treatment have serious side effects, including liver toxicity and heart rhythm problems, if taken with certain other drugs.

Unsightly fingernails and toenails from deforming fungus infections can deal a blow to one's vanity. They are ugly, and they keep getting uglier.

Several prescription medications are highly effective in stopping the infection, and they do it usually within a few months (three months for fingernails and up to six months for toenails). The drawback is the potential side effects of some of the medications. When given with the antibiotic erythromycin, the antihistamine Hismanal, and many other prescription and over-the-counter medications, they can cause severe, life-threatening heart rhythm disturbances.

Another side effect is life-threatening liver toxicity. The decision to use these drugs should be made by a patient who is aware of the possible side effects of the medication. Before starting these medications, you should discuss the pros and cons with your doctor.

•

Breast

Tip 45:

Any lump in the breast must be considered serious until proven otherwise.

Cancer of the breast is the most common cancer in women. Self-examination for a lump is the best way to detect this cancer early. Many lumps are harmless growths or are tiny balloonlike structures containing fluid, called cysts. But every lump should be evaluated by a doctor to rule out cancer.

It is important to remember that you can have a negative mammogram (a special X-ray of the breast) and still have cancer of the breast. Therefore the doctor should examine you first and try to locate the lump. Most women then obtain a mammogram. In young women (less than 40 years of age), the doctor may use a device called an ultrasound, which uses special sound waves to take a picture of the lump. The doctor may also insert a small needle to draw out any fluid or cells from the lump. For most women, examination of a piece of the lump (biopsy) under a microscope is the best way to make a definitive diagnosis of what is causing the abnormal growth.

Risk factors for breast cancer include a family history of breast cancer (especially in your mother or sisters, which puts you at a two-to-three-times-higher risk), increasing age (85 percent of breast cancers occur after the age of 40; half of all breast cancers occur in women over 65), obesity, a high-fat diet, exposure to radiation, a previous history of breast cancer, no children, having a baby at a late age (usually after 35), and going through menopause at a later age than normal (usually 45 to 55).

The key to beating breast cancer is early detection, which can best be achieved by following these American Cancer Society Guidelines:

1. Perform a breast self-exam every month during the week following your menstrual period. (See Appendix B for information on how to perform a breast self-exam.)
2. See your physician for a breast exam every year after age 40.
3. All women should obtain a baseline mammogram between 35 and 40 years of age. After 40, women should have a mammogram every year.

Contact your doctor immediately if you detect a lump in your breast.

Breast cancer rarely occurs in men, but any man with a breast lump should also be examined by a physician. One percent of all breast cancers occur in men.

> **Tip 46:**
>
> Changes in a breast: (1) redness and/or swelling,
> (2) dimpling of the skin, (3) orange peel appear-
> ance of the skin, (4) nipple retraction, or (5) crusty
> appearance of the nipple may indicate cancer even
> though you cannot feel a mass. Therefore a thor-
> ough medical evaluation is necessary as soon as
> possible.

If you were born with retracted nipples—nipples that
do not project outward—you may be unable to nurse
babies. Otherwise, you should have no problem related
to your nipples. But retraction of a previously normal
breast nipple may occur from a growth located under
the nipple and may be cancerous.

Deformities of the skin of the breast causing redness
or swelling, dimpling, an orange peel appearance,
and/or a crusty appearance of the nipples indicates progressive disease in the breast, which may be cancer.
These changes can be subtle, often occurring without
pain. But they are red light warning signals calling for
immediate medical evaluation.

> **Tip 47:**
>
> Three main types of fluids can drain abnor-
> mally from your breast nipple. The type of
> fluid is indicative of the underlying breast prob-
> lem.

Bloody discharge. A bloody discharge, sometimes watery and foul-smelling, from the nipple could be a serious matter. Most often, it originates from a localized growth (intraductal papilloma) in the lining of the tiny tube leading to the nipple of the breast. These tiny growths are so small that they cannot be felt by examining the breast. Although uncommon, intraductal cancer must be considered. A mammogram, biopsy, and/or surgical exploration of the nipple duct may be indicated to rule out cancer. See your doctor as soon as possible.

White milky fluid. A milky white substance leaking from one or both of your nipples is called galactorrhea.

Gently milk your nipple to see if you can draw out the fluid. Note the color, amount, and consistency. The fluid of galactorrhea has the consistency of water. The amount is usually small. It is similar to the fluid secreted during pregnancy.

The pituitary gland, which is attached to the undersurface of the brain, secretes prolactin, the hormone responsible for lactation. Certain benign (noncancerous) tumors of this gland oversecrete the substance, causing the breast to leak the white watery discharge. Other symptoms include absence or alteration of your menstrual periods and problems with your peripheral vision (loss of vision from the corners of your eyes). Tumors of this type are benign, but if untreated they can cause damage to surrounding brain structures, like the nerve of the eye.

Shingles (a painful rash caused by a virus), foreplay with the nipples, jogging without proper breast support, hypothyroidism (a low-functioning thyroid gland), and certain medications such as the major tranquilizers including Thorazine can also cause this nipple discharge. See your doctor for appropriate evaluation.

Green fluid. A green-colored, watery fluid coming from the nipple of one or both breasts is fairly common and usually benign, although it may persist. It is often noted by discovering a stain on your bra. You can make sure it is coming from the breast nipple by compressing the breast and noting the appearance of a drop of fluid on the nipple surface. Dab it with a tissue to note the color. The fluid often comes from small fluid-filled pockets in the breast caused by hormones. Your breasts may also be tender. It occurs usually around the time of menstruation, which is the time of maximum breast engorgement.

Tip 48:

Male breast enlargement commonly occurs in adolescents, obese persons, or alcohol drinkers. Also, certain medications can cause breast enlargement. It can be a sign of a hormonal imbalance. But on rare occasions it may be a sign of cancer in the testicles or lungs or of another serious ailment.

If you are an adult male and have noted an enlargement of your breasts, you may have a condition known as gynecomastia. The breast tissue is solid and lumpy, as opposed to the normal fat tissue near the nipples.

Some breast enlargement may be normal, resulting from higher levels of the hormone estrogen found in young developing boys or during puberty. As an adult, the hormone testosterone counteracts the effects of estrogen. Therefore normal adult men have very little breast tissue under their nipples.

The most common cause of abnormal breast enlargement is a side effect of medications, including diuretics, digitalis, Dilantin, the tuberculosis drug INH, spironolactone, methadone, anticancer drugs, some antihypertensive drugs, ketoconazole, cimetidine, theophylline, and Flagyl. These drugs can upset the balance of testosterone and estrogen. If possible, you and your doctor may decide to alter your medications. Anabolic steroids, alcohol, and marijuana have been reported to cause breast enlargement. In addition, elderly men sometimes develop gynecomastia because shrunken testicles result in reduced testosterone. Also, some men are born with Klinefelter's syndrome, which can lead to enlarged breast tissue and small testicles. This is reported to occur in one of every 500 men.

Less common causes of male breast enlargement include chronic liver disease, kidney disease, breast cancer, hypothyroidism, a pituitary gland tumor, and hormone-secreting tumors in organs such as the lungs and testicles. It is important that you seek medical evaluation to determine if you have any of these underlying ailments so that early treatment can be instituted.

Chest Area

Breathing Difficulties

Tip 49:

Difficulty breathing and a wheezing sound while breathing, often following physical exertion, are signs of an asthma attack. Left untreated, an asthma attack can lead to severe chest muscle fatigue and death.

How do you know when an asthma attack is life-threatening? The most important point is to note how long it lasts. Since asthma makes breathing difficult, it requires much more energy and therefore can lead to fatigue. The longer the attack goes on, the more tired you will get.

During an attack, as the muscles for breathing

become tired, the volume of air exchanged by the lungs will decrease. This decrease may be so subtle that you will hardly notice it. The result will be a drop in the oxygen level, accompanied by a rise in the carbon dioxide level in the blood.

Carbon dioxide is a by-product of body metabolism; it is carried by the bloodstream to the lungs, where it is exhaled out of the body. If the lungs cannot get rid of carbon dioxide, it will build up in your blood. A carbon dioxide buildup in the blood has a sedating effect on the brain, which may cause you to feel drowsy. You may lose the motivation or energy to breathe.

When respiratory failure develops, your condition may deteriorate rapidly. Death from respiratory arrest (cessation of breathing) can occur unexpectedly.

Urgent medical attention is necessary for a first-time asthma attack. Emergency medical care is also appropriate when an attack continues, does not improve, or gets worse. Signs that asthma is worsening include the need to use higher doses of inhalants, frequent episodes of shortness of breath (over two to three times per week), or decreasing peak flow measurements when using a special monitor device recommended by your doctor. Also, the signs of discomfort, such as struggling to breathe, may actually decrease from exhaustion, and if immediate medical intervention is not instituted, the person can die.

Tip 50:

Deformities of the chest can impair breathing and worsen over time.

Deformities of the chest are common birth defects that can affect the ability of the lungs to expand adequately. The chest wall is distorted, chest volume is reduced, and the heart may be displaced, encroaching on the lungs. There are three kinds of chest deformities that can interfere with breathing. Pectus excavatum is a sunken breastbone, scoliosis is a curved spine, and kyphoscoliosis is a hunchback condition with a curved spine. Kyphoscoliosis is the most common chest deformity that causes breathing problems.

As you get older, the muscles of the thorax may become weaker and further limit chest expansion, causing more serious breathing difficulties. Mild curvature of the spine may progress to a more serious stage, further distorting the chest.

These ailments increase the risk of developing pneumonia because the ability to cough up accumulated secretions is decreased and oxygen intake is limited.

If you have a chest deformity, have your lung function checked periodically by a physician. If you develop congestion, have it checked and treated right away.

Tip 51:

Excessive snoring and/or short episodes of "no breathing" during sleep, and daytime sleepiness may indicate that your oxygen supply is being cut off at night. This can result in serious health problems.

If you suffer from unexplained excessive daytime sleepiness (falling asleep at stoplights or while watching television) and you are told that you snore loudly or intermittently stop breathing when you sleep, then you may have a medical condition known as obstructive sleep apnea (OSA). OSA is more often seen in African Americans and obese adults with short necks and floppy airways. During sleep part of the back of the roof of the mouth (soft palate), the tonsils, or the base of the tongue is flip-flopping over your airway, causing you to snore and intermittently stop breathing for a few seconds. You may wake up but not know why. The impact of intermittently cutting the oxygen supply to the body has serious consequences: high blood pressure and permanent damage to the brain, heart, and lungs.

The diagnosis of OSA can be made by special tests ordered by your physician. Treatment often includes the use of a breathing assist device, called a C-PAP, while sleeping. The C-PAP pushes air through a mask you wear to keep your airway open. In some selected cases surgery may also be indicated to correct the problem.

Go on a diet if you are overweight. Avoid alcoholic beverages and sedative medications, which can worsen the condition, and don't drive until the problem is corrected. This condition is an emergency if you stop breathing more than once every two minutes or you stop breathing for more than one minute at a time. The sooner you are evaluated and treated, the less the risk of serious complications.

Tip 52:

Shortness of breath may indicate a serious heart or lung disease or a very low blood count (anemia).

In simple terms, your lungs are like trees. The trunk and branches, however, are not filled with wood but are actually tubes filled with air (see Figure 4). At the end of each branch are "balloons." When you inhale, the air travels from the trunk of the tree through all the various branches and fills the balloons (the medical term is alveoli) with oxygen. When you exhale, the balloons deflate, and carbon dioxide passes through the branches, then through the trunk and out of your mouth and nose. Very small blood vessels, called capillaries, run near these tiny balloons. At the site where these tiny blood vessels and balloons touch each other, the red blood cells flowing through the vessels load up with oxygen and get rid of carbon dioxide.

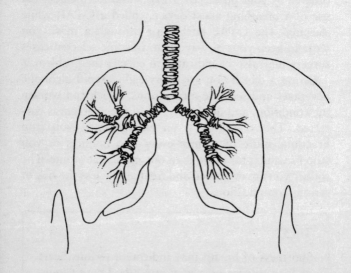

Figure 4. Lungs.

The various causes of shortness of breath require completely different therapies. Many causes are either a result of swelling or blockage of the tubes carrying air to and from the lungs, or a result of a problem at the site where the alveoli and blood vessels exchange gases. Shortness of breath can also be the result of weakened breathing muscles or nerves.

In many instances the doctor's first step is to give you oxygen through a mask. The second step is to treat the underlying ailment.

Many problems occur at the site of the tubes. Food can get stuck there, requiring instant emergency measures: the Heimlich maneuver. (See the section on "Choking" in Appendix A.) The tubes can swell from causes such as allergies, dust, and infections. Bronchitis (infection in the tubes) is treated with antibiotics, while asthma (swelling of the tubes often caused by allergies) is treated with various medications to decrease the swelling and open the tubes.

On the other hand, if the disease is at the site of the alveoli and blood vessels, other therapies may be necessary. For example, blood clots in the vessels require a blood thinner. A shortage of red blood cells, which carry the oxygen, may indicate the need for a blood transfusion. A weak heart (heart failure) may cause a backup of fluid into the lungs; this condition may require a medication to strengthen the pumping action of the heart (like digoxin) or to rid the body of excess fluids (like a diuretic). Also, a partial or total blockage in the heart's arteries (angina or heart attack) can sometimes cause shortness of breath on exertion without chest pain (see Tips 66 and 69). Pneumonia causes an accumulation of bacteria or viruses, white blood cells, and other by-products of infection, which clog up the vessels and alveoli.

If you are merely breathing too rapidly and your

tubes, alveoli, and vessels are in good working order, you may be hyperventilating. This condition can be associated with headache, light-headedness, blurry vision, muscle spasms and numbness, and tingling around the mouth and hands. When you hyperventilate, too much carbon dioxide is exhaled. The resulting change in your body chemistry makes you feel that you have to breathe even more, and thus the condition worsens. Many things, including frightening situations, mouth breathing, fatigue, and repeated sighs can trigger hyperventilation. Frequent sighing and yawning may be a sign of long-term hyperventilation related to underlying anxiety.

The doctor can determine the cause of your shortness of breath by performing different procedures and tests, including listening to your lungs, checking the oxygen and red blood cell count in your blood, and taking various pictures of your lungs (X-rays, scans, etc.).

Shortness of breath might be a symptom of a serious heart or lung disease that could require urgent medical attention because the lack of oxygen in the body can cause all parts of your body to fail. Getting the proper amount of oxygen into your lungs and correcting the underlying problem is very important. Since shortness of breath can be the sign of a life-threatening condition, immediate medical evaluation is appropriate.

Tip 53:

If you suddenly get short of breath after injuring your leg, you may have a blood clot in your lung. You need to be taken to an emergency room immediately.

A blow to your leg can damage the wall of a vein and cause the blood in the vein to clot. The swelling from the injury can also slow blood flow in the vein, causing clots to form. Pieces of the clot can flow up the bloodstream to the lung. You are in need of emergency therapy to thin the blood, possibly dissolve the clot or remove it. Immediate treatment can save your life.

Tip 54:

If you develop a cough and/or shortness of breath after surgery, even a week or two afterward, you may have a blood clot in your lung, or pneumonia. You may first have noticed swelling and tenderness in the back of your lower leg or in your groin. This is where the clot originated before traveling in the veins to your lung.

During and after surgery, especially in the belly area or on the bones and joints, you are at a high risk of developing blood clots in the veins of your pelvis and legs. This is because blood flow slows down in these areas. If a fragment of the clot breaks off and flows up the bloodstream to the lungs, you may experience sudden shortness of breath, chest pain on taking a deep breath, and a cough.

For this reason it is very important to notify your doctor immediately if you notice swelling and tenderness in your groin or leg at any time including after surgery, even a week or two after you have gone home. Also, you are more susceptible to developing infections, such as pneumonia, after surgery. Pneumonia can cause shortness of breath, cough, and a fever. In both cases you need emergency evaluation and therapy.

Tip 55:

If you smoke and find it difficult to breathe, you may have an advanced form of emphysema, which could eventually kill you. You are also more likely to have an infection or lung cancer.

Shortness of breath in a smoker can be the first sign of emphysema, cancer of the lung, heart disease, or pneumonia, to which smokers are more susceptible.

Emphysema, most often caused by smoking, can lead to permanent lung failure and eventually death. Therefore knowing you have emphysema might be a stimulus to stop smoking.

Emphysema traps air in the microscopic air sacs that make up the lungs. When air enters into them, it has trouble getting out due to the spasm and destruction of the wall of the tiny air passages that lead to the air sac, and due to secretions in the air passages prompted by irritation from smoke. As a result, the tiny air sacs become overinflated, and they no longer empty their contents when air is exhaled. This leaves a considerable amount of dead air (air poor in oxygen) in them, instead of a full load of fresh air with each breath. These sacs are where the body normally obtains its oxygen for the blood, so a reduction of available oxygen in the air sacs reduces the body's supply.

At first, you may not notice that your breathing is becoming impaired. Long before abnormalities appear on a chest X-ray or you have difficulty breathing, changes can be detected with lung function testing.

Lung function testing involves breathing into a machine that makes several measurements, including the total lung volume as well as the rate of airflow in and out of the lungs. The earliest measurement for diagnosing emphysema is the amount of air exhaled from the lung during the first second.

If you smoke, ask your doctor for a lung function test, and pay attention to the results. Stop smoking—it could save your life. If you smoke and are short of breath, it is necessary that you see a doctor immediately to rule out emphysema, pneumonia, lung cancer, and other ailments.

Tip 56:

Shortness of breath when you lie flat in bed, which wakes you up in the middle of the night and improves when you sit up, is often a sign of heart failure.

The heart is one big muscle that pumps blood through your body. If the pump begins to fail, fluid can back up into your lungs and cause shortness of breath. In the earlier stages of heart failure, the shortness of breath comes only when you exercise, climb stairs, or walk uphill. It also occurs when you are lying flat in bed or sleeping on one pillow.

The reason is related to a shift in the fluid in your body. When you are erect or sitting, the fluid accumulates in the dependent parts of your body—the lower legs and feet. Often, people with heart failure who have excess fluid have swelling of their legs, ankles, and feet during the day when they are in an upright position. This may go unnoticed because it produces no discomfort. But, when you are lying flat, the fluid from your legs is returned to the circulation and to the heart, which is too weak to pump it all, causing the fluid to shift to the lungs.

The scientific name for this condition is PND (paroxysmal nocturnal dyspnea), which means shortness of breath at night that occurs intermittently. You go to sleep, awaken short of breath, sit up and breathe better, then lie back down and get short of breath again. You may eventually use two or three pillows to sleep on. If the condition is bad enough, you may have to sit up in a chair all night.

There are many causes of heart failure. When any symptoms of heart failure appear, including nighttime shortness of breath, it is urgent that the cause be found. Evaluation and treatment can be lifesaving.

Tip 57:

Sudden shortness of breath, especially if accompanied by chest pain and a cough with bloody phlegm, can mean you have a blood clot in your lung. Tumors and certain pneumonias can also cause these symptoms. You need emergency evaluation and treatment.

A blood clot in the lung occurs when a clot in a vein (often in a leg) breaks apart and a piece of it travels through the blood vessels into the lung. The clot may also originate in the right chamber of the heart. If the clot is small, a small area of the lung will be damaged. However, a large clot may follow, which can damage a larger area and may even be fatal. The formation of a clot may take several days or may occur rapidly over a few hours. When the breakoff occurs, however, it takes only seconds for the piece to travel to your lung.

Anyone who has had surgery or who has been sitting for a long period of time (such as while traveling by car or airplane) is more likely to develop a blood clot in a leg, often with tenderness and swelling in the back of the lower leg. Clots also often develop in the veins inside the pelvic area, with tenderness and swelling in the groin. This problem may not be noticeable and may not appear until after the hospitalized patient is home. Shortness of breath may be the first sign that something is wrong.

An injury to the leg can also cause blood to clot in a leg vein, where it can travel to the lung. On the other hand, injuries to the leg usually cause blood to flow out of the injured blood vessels into the tissue and then form large bruises or pockets of blood called hematomas. They pose little threat, since blood that clots outside the blood vessels goes nowhere.

Certain diseases can cause blood to clot more readily. Birth control pills may also increase blood clotting and, if possible, should be avoided if you have a prior history of blood clots. Pregnancy also increases your chances of developing a blood clot.

If you have had a blood clot, you are at a higher risk of having them again. Blood clots are life-threatening and require emergency therapy.

Tumors in the lung and certain pneumonias (including those caused by bacteria and tuberculosis) are some of the other ailments that can cause shortness of breath, chest pain, and a bloody cough. If you develop any of these red light warning signals, get to an emergency room immediately.

> **Tip 58:**
>
> If you get more shortness of breath than normal
> with mild exertion, often accompanied by a more
> rapid pulse, you may have a serious medical
> problem, usually in your lungs or heart.

Normally you get short of breath and your heart
speeds up when you exert yourself, such as when you
run up a flight of stairs. But if your shortness of breath
and/or rapid pulse continue too long after rest (usually
three minutes or more), or if they occur with very mild
exertion, then you may have a heart-lung problem, a
low blood count, or another serious illness. Immediate
medical evaluation and therapy are appropriate.

> **Tip 59:**
>
> Wheezing means you potentially have a serious
> lung problem.

Wheezing is the noise produced by air as it is forced
through narrowed air passages in the lung when
you breathe out. Narrowing of the air passages
may suddenly occur due to a squeezing of the muscles
(bronchospasm) in the wall of the small airways.
This produces asthma, and it may be the result of
an allergic reaction (see Tip 160), an inhaled irritant, or
a reaction to medicines, stress, and inhaling cold air.

Asthma attacks can be severe and life-threatening. Even if your wheezing has been only mild, you could have an attack so severe that you would not be able to breathe. Therefore, if you wheeze, you should be evaluated for asthma. The treatment includes sprays and pills that can relax the muscles in the walls of the airways.

Emphysema can also cause wheezing by destroying lung tissue, which results in narrowed air passages in the lungs. In emphysema there are also pockets of dead air space in the lungs, due to destruction of the tiny air sacs. This stale air takes up space in the lungs, limiting the amount of fresh air you can breathe in. Therefore you don't get enough oxygen in your blood. If the disease progresses, it can be fatal.

Tumors in the lung can also block air passages and cause wheezing.

Smoking can destroy your lungs by worsening asthma and causing emphysema and tumors. If you smoke, *stop!* Consult your doctor for assistance. If you wheeze, it is important that you are medically evaluated as soon as possible to determine the cause and appropriate therapy.

•

Cough

Tip 60:

Coughing up blood may be a sign of bronchitis, pneumonia, blood clots, or cancer.

If you are coughing up blood, it is important to find out where the blood is originating. A small amount of blood from bleeding gums, a nosebleed, or a cut on your mouth may trickle down and irritate your throat, causing you to cough it up. Or the bleeding may actually originate in your lungs, which suggests the presence of blood clots or an infection, possibly tuberculosis. Also, you may have an abnormal growth in your lungs, possibly cancer. You need to see a doctor immediately for evaluation and appropriate therapy.

A thorough examination of your mouth and nose, and even looking into your lung with a tube, may determine the cause of the bleeding. X-rays and scans of your lungs may also be helpful.

Tip 61:

Coughing up dirty-looking phlegm may mean that there is pus in it from an infection.

When you get a cold or the flu, you usually cough up phlegm. It is important to note the color. Mucus produced by the lungs, airways, nose, and sinuses is usually clear and often thicker than water.

Mucous production can be primed by allergies, irritants like cigarette smoke, or illnesses like a cold and the flu. "Dirty-looking" phlegm, usually gray or green, contains pus cells, which may come from a lung infection like bronchitis or pneumonia. When the infection is confined to the air passages, you have bronchitis. When it invades the substance of the lung, you have pneumonia. These infections may be caused by a number of different germs, including certain bacteria that require antibiotics or viruses that resolve without taking antibiotics. Also, smokers, diabetics, or people with other serious medical problems may require antibiotics.

When the phlegm turns dirty, seek medical evaluation and treatment, especially if fever and fatigue are present or if you have other medical ailments. The doctor will determine what type of infection is present and, if the infection is caused by bacteria, the most effective antibiotic for treatment.

Tip 62:

A persistent cough lasting over two weeks may indicate tuberculosis, pneumonia, bronchitis, heart disease, or cancer. Reflux of stomach contents into the esophagus (the tube between the mouth and the stomach) can cause an annoying cough. On rare occasions, food and acid may reflux from the stomach into the windpipe, damaging your lungs over time. Certain medicines can also cause a nagging cough.

Everyone coughs from time to time, whether from postnasal drip, a cold, an allergy, or irritants in the air. Most of these minor illnesses will run their course in fourteen days or less. If a cough lasts longer or if it is associated with additional symptoms, other causes must be considered by a physician. Some of these are life-threatening. They include a lung infection, heart disease, or cancer. Smokers often cough constantly, so they may not realize that a more serious disease is present.

When routine treatments for coughs have failed, and more traditional causes of coughs have been ruled out, another possibility is a reflux of stomach contents into the esophagus, which can be associated with a hiatal hernia. A hiatal hernia is when part of the stomach pokes through a hole in the diaphragm, which separates the chest from the abdomen. This condition can wake you up at night with the feeling that you are strangling. You might cough so hard that it takes your breath away, and you black out. A hiatal hernia or other conditions can allow acid-containing fluid to back up the esophagus and then into the windpipe causing spasm and a cough. This is called acid reflux.

Acid liquid can flow up the esophagus much more easily when you are lying down, so the reflux occurs most often at night. When the liquid enters the windpipe, it can irritate the lining, which can cause repeated coughing episodes throughout the day and night.

If the cause of your cough is a hiatal hernia, you need to take medication for your stomach problem, not an antibiotic or cold medicine for your cough. If your lungs become soiled by acid over a long period of time, scarring may occur, along with a reduction in lung function.

Treatment begins with prescription medicines designed to suppress acid formation in the stomach. Other practical measures are important as well. Before lying down, remain upright for at least an hour after eating or drinking. Avoid overeating at any time. Elevate the head of your bed by placing a brick under the legs at the head. This will raise the head of the bed four inches—enough of an incline to reduce the acid reflux yet not disturb sleep.

Long-term coughing may also be a result of asthma and postnasal drip, which also need to be ruled out as causes by your doctor. In addition, a chronic cough may also be a side effect of medications, including a class of blood pressure and heart medications known as ACE inhibitors. If you take one of these blood pressure pills and have a cough, tell your doctor.

Tip 63:

A cough, fever, and chest pains with or without other common cold symptoms are sometimes indicators of blood clots in the lungs (see Tips 52 to 54) and often of pneumonia. Failure to improve after forty-eight hours of treatment for pneumonia is a strong indication of a more serious infection requiring immediate medical evaluation.

Often people think pneumonia always follows a bad "cold." That is, first you have the typical cold symptoms—congestion in the head and a sore throat that then spreads to the chest with coughing. Not so. The first symptoms may be the sudden onset of a cough, fever, and chest pains, with no cold symptoms whatsoever. If this occurs, you should see your doctor right away.

Once you start treatment for pneumonia, your condition should improve within forty-eight hours. If it does not, touch base with your doctor again. Seek immediate medical attention if you develop shortness of breath, since the therapy may be ineffective and the infection can spread rapidly. It may indicate that the infection in your lungs is at a very serious stage.

Pneumonia is often caused by the bacterium pneumococcus in senior citizens and in frail or disabled persons. The vaccine for pneumococcal pneumonia may prevent the disease or help the body's defenses fight it.

Many other germs cause pneumonia, including staphylococcus, mycoplasma, and hemophilus. An odd germ causes Legionnaires' disease, which is difficult to culture and identify. The illness starts with nonspecific aching and diarrhea. It infects the lungs and can bring about rapid death if not treated. The secret to survival is early diagnosis and appropriate antibiotic treatment. The disease is named Legionnaires' disease because it was first discovered at an American Legion conference. Several members of the American Legion contracted the disease where the germ had contaminated the conference room's air-conditioning system.

If the cough, fever, and chest pain are diagnosed as being due to blood clots in the lung, your doctor will start you on blood thinners and other therapies immediately. Treatment can be lifesaving.

Tip 64:

Cough, fever, and night sweats may be signs of tuberculosis.

For a while tuberculosis (TB) seemed to be a disease of the past. Improved medications and the isolation of

infected persons helped decrease the prevalence of
this ailment. But stronger forms of the bacterium
have caused a marked resurgence of TB. Even power-
ful drugs are not as effective in killing these new TB
germs.

TB infections most commonly occur in the lungs
but can spread to other parts of the body. A cough is
often an early symptom. Tuberculosis is usually accompanied by weight loss, an overall ill feeling, and night
sweats.

TB can spread through nursing homes, attacking
senior citizens, the debilitated, and AIDS patients.
But there are also outbreaks of TB among healthy individuals. These outbreaks are more likely to occur in
close quarters where air is recirculated through air-
conditioning systems.

Fever, cough, and night sweats warrant immediate
evaluation by a physician. If you have tuberculosis,
adhere to your medical regimen, since the disease can be
fatal. In addition to tuberculosis, other causes of these
symptoms are other infections of the lung and cancers
such as lymphoma.

Tip 65:

If you have a smokers' cough, you are at
much higher risk of developing a serious lung
infection.

Tobacco smoke irritates the entire respiratory system, including the nose, sinuses, throat, windpipe,
and lungs. This irritation injures the surface of these

areas, reducing their ability to remove mucus secretions and defend against germ invasion. These changes lead to more frequent infections of the nose, sinuses, throat, and lungs. Damage to the mucous lining causes persistent congestion and coughing, which is a prime setup for developing pneumonia. A chronic cough may hide a lung infection or other serious lung ailments.

Reduce your risk of developing serious infections. Stop smoking. You will also feel better.

•

Chest Pain and Chest Discomfort

Tip 66:

Recognize the chest discomfort of a heart attack. Emergency medical care can save your life.

The pain and tightness of a heart attack occurs classically in the center or left side of the chest under the breastbone. The pain may extend into the inner aspect of the left arm, stopping at the elbow. Common variations in the locale of this pain are near the front base of the neck, or in the jaw (see Figure 5). The arm pain may not occur.

The character of the pain can be crushing or pressure-like, also described as a constricting or squeezing feeling. It often resembles indigestion, and it feels as though

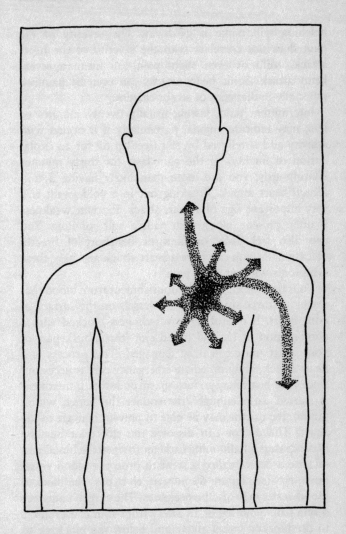

Figure 5. Chest Pain Warning of a Possible Heart Attack.

belching will make it go away. The severity of the pain does not correlate with the severity of the heart attack. Mild or even slight pain can mean a severe heart attack. Some heart attacks can even be painless, especially in diabetics or senior citizens.

Intermittent pain, lasting usually twenty minutes or less, may indicate angina, particularly if it occurs with activity and is relieved by rest (see Tip 69 for an explanation of angina). If the pain lasts for thirty minutes continuously, you are more than likely having a full-blown heart attack. Breaking out in a cold sweat is a very important sign of a heart attack. Extreme weakness is often present, along with nausea and vomiting. You can also feel dizzy or faint or be short of breath. Occasionally, you can have a heart attack and have these symptoms without chest pain.

Your heart itself requires nourishment from blood that travels in three small but vital vessels on the surface of your heart. If one of these vessels gets blocked with a combination of fat and blood clot (thrombus), part of your heart muscle will be damaged. This process is a heart attack, and immediate emergency care is necessary since your heart may go into spasm and stop. If treatment is started early enough (the sooner the better, within hours), the doctor may be able to prevent damage to the heart. The doctor can dissolve the clot (clot busters) and/or insert a ballooning catheter to open the blood vessel, use a device called a stent to prop the blood vessel open, etc. (see Figure 6). Surgery to bypass the blocked blood vessel may also be necessary. The surgeon attaches a vein from your leg or an artery from your chest muscle to the blocked vessel above and below the blockage so blood can flow around it. Sometimes treatment with medicines alone is indicated.

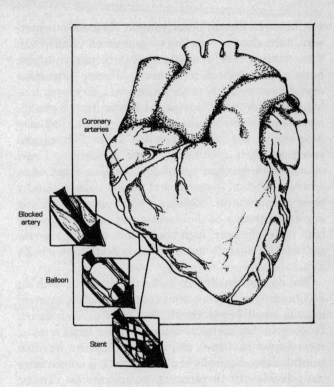

Figure 6. Heart.

Tip 67:

There are unusual presentations of a heart attack, such as a painless heart attack. Awareness can save your life.

A heart attack can occur without chest pain or pressure in the chest or a feeling of indigestion (see Tip 85). Even without these symptoms it can be just as deadly, but it is more difficult to diagnose. You may experience any or a combination of the following: a very weak feeling, sudden dizziness, a feeling that your heart is pounding, shortness of breath, or a heavy sweat. You may have only a feeling of impending doom. Nausea and vomiting often accompany these symptoms. Heart attacks without chest discomfort are seen more often among diabetics, women, and senior citizens. Under these circumstances, consider a heart attack, especially if you have other cardiovascular risk factors including high blood pressure, high cholesterol, obesity, a smoking habit, or a family history of early death from a heart attack.

The doctor usually can make the diagnosis with an EKG and "dye" (intravenous contrast) studies, examining the small blood vessels that nourish your heart. Blood tests for chemical changes in the heart muscle, special types of X-rays, and scans of the heart are often helpful. Early diagnosis of a heart attack is crucial since its possible life-threatening complications can be treated. In certain instances immediate therapy can prevent permanent heart damage.

Tip 68:

If you think you are having a heart attack with symptoms such as chest pain, chew one regular, full-strength aspirin immediately unless you are allergic to aspirin. It could save your life. Also, get to an emergency room immediately.

It may seem ridiculous to take something as simple as an aspirin for something as serious as a heart attack, but it does help prevent damage to the heart muscle during a heart attack.

Your heart has three small but vital blood vessels on its surface. These arteries provide blood to nourish the heart muscle itself. As fatty substances such as cholesterol clog up the vessels, eventually only a small amount of blood can pass through. It is like a small pea stuck in a straw, with only a little opening around the pea.

This is a perfect setting for a blood clot to form, which can completely block the artery. It ultimately causes the heart attack, because no blood can pass through to provide oxygen and nourishment to the heart muscle. Part of your heart muscle is damaged, and you develop chest pain. Depending on the location and size of the damage to the heart, different things can happen: The heart may beat irregularly, the heart may become weak and lose its pumping strength, or the heart may even stop pumping altogether.

Aspirin (not Tylenol or other pain medications) actually "unsticks" the components of the blood known as platelets, which help form the clot. If you chew an aspirin when you initially feel chest pain, the blood clot may partially dissolve or at least may stop forming. Some blood will then be able to pass around the fatty blockage and therefore continue to deliver oxygen to the heart muscle, preventing a more serious heart attack.

> **Tip 69:**
>
> If you have chest pain, tightness, and burning, extending to the neck, throat, jaw, and/or left shoulder and upper arm, usually lasting less than twenty minutes, often occurring with exertion but sometimes during rest or sleep, you may be experiencing angina. Angina is due to insufficient blood flow to the heart muscle. It is often a precursor to a heart attack and needs immediate evaluation and treatment.

Your heart muscle has three small but vital blood vessels on its surface. When one or more of these blood vessels becomes partially blocked, the heart muscle does not get enough oxygen and nutrition. Subsequent changes in the heart muscle irritate its nerve supply, producing pain.

Typically angina presents itself as chest pain, tightness, and burning, which can extend to the neck, throat, jaw, and/or left shoulder and upper arm. The pain usually lasts less than twenty minutes and never longer than thirty minutes. Sometimes the discomfort is not in the chest but is only in the neck, throat, jaw, left shoulder, or upper arm. It often appears when you exert yourself, either mildly or more strenuously, while shaving, walking upstairs, lifting objects, or exercising. The pain disappears with the cessation of exertion. It can also occur without exertion.

Angina differs from a heart attack in that the artery supplying the heart muscle is not totally blocked by fat or blood clots. In a heart attack the blockage is total.

The lack of oxygen and nutrition persists, the chest pain continues, and part of the heart muscle is irreversibly damaged.

If you have angina, you are at a higher risk of having a heart attack. The partially blocked artery, which is responsible for causing your angina, is easily susceptible to total blockage by a blood clot. Anyone having angina attacks should have a thorough heart evaluation, which usually includes an EKG while exercising and a catheterization to examine the arteries that nourish the heart.

There are many effective medical treatments for angina. It is urgent that you go to the emergency room in the following situations, which may be red light warning signals of an impending heart attack:

1. The first time you notice you have angina
2. Angina when you are at rest
3. Angina that wakes you up at night
4. A change in the pattern of your angina pain, such as becoming more severe, more frequent, or longer lasting

---

Tip 70:

If your father, mother, brother, or sister died at a young age (men before 50, women before 60) from a heart attack, you need to be checked for risk factors even if you are only in your twenties.

The early death of an immediate family member from a heart attack is a warning sign that you are at a higher risk of having one. Taking the following actions can decrease your risk: (1) reduce fat intake in your diet; (2) stop smoking; (3) seek treatment if you have high blood pressure; (4) exercise regularly; (5) adjust your lifestyle to reduce stress; (6) diet with the advice of a dietitian if you are overweight; and (7) see your doctor for cardiac risk factor screening.

Tip 71:

Severe, prolonged chest pain under the breast-bone that extends to the back between the shoul-der blades is uncommon but may indicate a rare life-threatening condition.

This type of pain is the classic pain pattern of a dissecting aneurysm of the thoracic aorta. The thoracic aorta, the huge artery that comes out of the heart, is the main thoroughfare in the distribution of blood to all parts of the body. The aortic wall is made up of three layers and is constantly subjected to pulsating pressure from the heartbeat, especially when the blood pressure is too high. This kind of stress can weaken and tear the inner layer of the wall, which allows blood to work its way into the wall itself and cause the lay-ers to separate (dissection). This weakened wall can also balloon out. (The ballooning out is called an aneurysm.)

This condition constitutes a true medical emergency. You need to be taken to an emergency room as quickly as possible. If the aneurysm ruptures through the outer wall of the aorta, massive bleeding and death will follow.

Other possible causes of this type of pain include a stomach ulcer that has broken through the stomach wall, pancreas inflammation, or gallbladder disease. All of these conditions warrant immediate medical evaluation. There are inherited disorders that increase your chance of having an aortic aneurysm. If you have a family member with an aortic aneurysm, you need to be evaluated.

Tip 72:

A sudden sharp pain on the side of your chest with shortness of breath may indicate a collapsed lung (pneumothorax). This and some other causes of these symptoms (see Tip 52) need emergency treatment.

When you breathe in, your lungs are full of air, and they still contain air when you breathe out. If there is a leak of air from the surface of the lung into the chest cavity, this leaked air can collapse the lung. You will experience a sudden, sharp pain on the side of the chest when the lung collapses. Shortness of breath follows.

A common cause of a collapsed lung is the bursting of a weakened area on the lung's surface. A small balloon-like area (called a bleb) on the surface of the lung ruptures. You may be born with such a weak spot, but it usually will not rupture until late adolescence or adulthood. It occurs more commonly in tall thin young men, often during exertion. Recurrence is frequent because those who have one weak spot on the lung often have many. A weak spot on the lung can also rupture in a patient with emphysema who smokes. It can occur whenever the chest wall is punctured, such as in an accident. Air gets into the chest cavity, which presses on and collapses the lung.

A collapsed lung constitutes a medical emergency, especially if the remaining lung is diseased. If the other organs in the chest, including the heart and major blood vessels, shift their position because of the lung collapse, they may encroach on the remaining lung. Emergency treatment is necessary to reexpand the collapsed lung because this condition can compromise the function of the other lung, leading to breathing failure and death.

Tip 73:

Pain under the breastbone after a vomiting episode, especially if bright red blood is vomited, may indicate a tear in the esophagus.

The esophagus is the muscular tube that takes food from the throat, through the chest, to the stomach. Food does not just fall through the tube; it is moved along by a wave of muscles in the wall of the esophagus, which squeeze the food through the tube. When vomiting occurs, the reverse happens. The stomach contracts, moving material into the esophagus, where the esophagus grabs it and, with a reversed wave of muscle contraction, hurls it out of the mouth. During episodes of severe vomiting, squeezing of the muscle wall of the esophagus can be profound, sufficient to tear the lining of the lower esophagus near the opening to the stomach. A life-threatening hemorrhage or infection may follow.

The wall of the esophagus can also weaken. Continued vomiting may lead to rupture, which is rapidly fatal. Early signs of this condition indicate the need for emergency medical treatment.

Tip 74:

Tenderness and pain in the back of your lower leg, and/or chest pain, and/or shortness of breath, occurring after sitting for a long time (as on a long trip), or after lying in bed for an extended period of time, are symptoms of a potentially dangerous blood clot.

A blood clot can form in your leg during a long trip in a car or airplane or when you are bedridden even for a short time. The sitting and lying positions cause more pooling of blood in the legs than does standing. When your legs are still, lack of leg muscle activity results in less blood flowing uphill from the legs. The blood that pools in your legs is more likely to clot. The leg, usually at the level of the calf, gets swollen, painful, and tender to touch (see Figure 7). If this occurs and if you suddenly develop chest pain or get short of breath, a piece of a clot in your leg may have broken off and traveled through the bloodstream to your lungs. You need to be taken to an emergency room immediately, because this condition can cause life-threatening damage to your lungs.

This condition can often be prevented if, during a

long trip, you take short walks to break up the sitting, by walking around the airplane or stopping the car for a break. If you are bedridden, taking short walks, if possible, may prevent the formation of blood clots. (See Tip 131 for other causes of blood clots to form in the leg.)

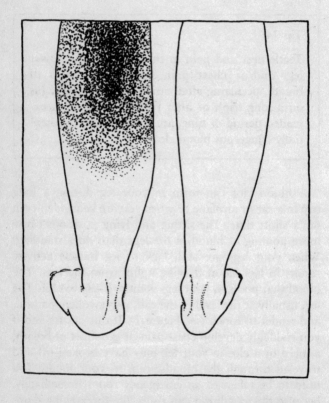

Figure 7. Leg Pain Location Which May Indicate a Blood Clot.

Tip 75:

Chest pain that gets worse when you take a deep breath (pleurisy) may indicate a blood clot, pneumonia, injury to the chest wall, a collapsed lung, a tumor in the lung, or other lung diseases.

Pleurisy is not a disease but a symptom. It is an irritation of the membrane (pleura) that lines the walls of the chest and the surface of the lung. The pleura is very smooth, slick, and moist, so as to decrease the friction between the lung and the chest wall during the expansion and deflation of the breathing cycle. If the pleura becomes irritated, swollen, or roughened from any disease process, a sharp, stabbing pain will often occur as the lung and the chest wall rub against each other during breathing.

Pleurisy makes you feel as though your breath is being cut off. Pneumonia, a common cause, involves the tissue near the surface of your lung, from which the inflammation may spread to the pleura and cause pleurisy. But it is possible to have pneumonia without having pleurisy.

A blood clot in the lung, a viral infection, a growth in the lung, an injury to the chest wall, a collapsed lung, lupus, and other diseases affecting the lungs may also cause pleurisy if the lining of the lung is inflamed.

Emergency medical evaluation and therapy are necessary.

Tip 76:

Chest pain that is worse when you are lying down but gets better when you sit up and bend forward may be caused by inflammation of the sac that holds the heart. Subsequently fluid may accumulate in the sac, squeezing the heart and interfering with its pumping.

The heart is contained in a saclike structure called the pericardium. This compartment is located in the left side of the chest, and if inflamed, it will cause pain in that area. Inflammation (swelling and irritation) of this sac is usually caused by a viral infection. It can also occur from a bacterial infection, from the spread of a cancerous growth from the lung, from waste products in the blood when the kidneys fail, and after a heart attack or certain heart surgeries. Also, certain medications (procainamide, hydralazine, the tuberculosis medicine isoniazid), can cause a lupus-type disease that can result in inflammation of the pericardium.

The chest pain produced by this condition (called pericarditis) may be similar to pain from pleurisy, pneumonia, or even a heart attack. The special characteristic of pericarditis is that the pain is often worse when you lie flat on your back. Sitting up and bending forward can ease the pain by relieving the pressure on the sac that contains the heart. Occasionally the chest pain varies in other ways with changes in position. This does not mean that you absolutely have pericarditis.

A potential complication of this disease is the weeping of fluid from the sac wall into the compartment around the heart. If a large amount of this fluid accumulates, it can compress the heart so it cannot effectively pump blood throughout the body, resulting in a failure of other organs in the body. This is referred to as cardiac tamponade. It is important to have pericarditis diagnosed immediately so you can receive treatment and/or close monitoring of the ailment.

•

Irregular Heartbeats and Heart Sounds

Tip 77:

If you have rapid, slow, or irregular heartbeat the red light warning signals may be: heart palpitations, fluttering, skipped beats, flopping beats, sudden spells of weakness, sudden spells of dizziness, "squirrels running around in the chest," and heart pounding. If you think your heart is beating abnormally fast, slow, or irregular, take your pulse. An abnormal pulse can be a warning sign of many different life-threatening illnesses.

If you feel that your heart is beating abnormally fast, as if it is racing and pounding in your chest, or is beating too slowly, or is beating with an irregular rhythm, take your pulse. To do so, take the pads of your second and third fingers, place them on the thumb side of your wrist, and find the pulsations of the artery. If your hand

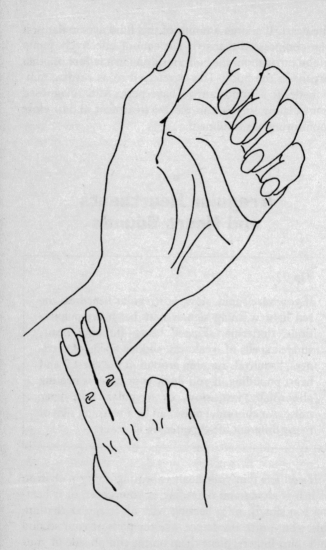

Figure 8. Taking a Pulse.

is palm up, the pulse is between the bone and the first big tendon (see Figure 8).

Count the number of pulsations you feel in one minute:

- A normal rate is usually between 60 and 100 beats per minute. Normal ranges of resting rates vary from person to person. In other words, if your normal rate is 60 to 70, an abnormally high rate for you may be 90. Or if a normal resting rate for you is 85 to 95, then an abnormally slow rate might be 60. It is a good idea to check your pulse a few times while at rest and get to know the general range of your pulse.
- A fast rate is a rate above your normal resting rate. A resting rate above 100 is abnormal for anyone.
- A resting heart rate is considered slow when it is below your normal range. For almost everybody, a rate below 60 beats per minute is slow.

It is normal for your pulse rate to rise as high as 120 with exercise, emotional change, fatigue, or fever. It may slow down during sleep. It can also be influenced by certain medications.

A rapid pulse can be the body's red light warning signal of a life-threatening internal hemorrhage (usually accompanied by weakness and dizziness when you are going from a lying position to a sitting position, or from a sitting position to a standing position).

In young, healthy people, irregular heartbeats are due to a small amount of abnormal electrical activity in a part of the heart. This occurs in about 20 percent of the young population. It can be brought on by stress, caffeine, or alcohol. Sometimes there is no explanation. These events are usually harmless and often go away when the heart speeds up during or after exercise.

Irregular, fast, and slow pulses can be dangerous and require immediate therapy in an emergency room. Examples of some of the more common causes are listed in Tips 78 through 83.

Tip 78:

A rapid pulse may appear with the following symptoms: heart palpitations, fluttering, skipped beats, flopping beats, sudden spells of weakness, sudden spells of dizziness, and/or heart pounding. A persistent rise in your pulse may be a sign that you are bleeding, often in the stomach or intestines. Emergency medical treatment can be lifesaving.

A rise in pulse may be a signal of a life-threatening hemorrhage in areas such as the stomach or intestines. Before the blood pressure drops, a rising pulse may be the first sign that bleeding is taking place. There are other causes of a rapid pulse, including a fever or side effects of certain medications.

Tip 79:

The sudden onset of a rapid pulse, especially if it starts and stops intermittently, may appear with the following symptoms: heart palpitations, fluttering, skipped beats, flopping beats, sudden spells of weakness and/or dizziness, and/or heart pounding. The intermittent rapid pulse is most likely caused by an abnormality in the electrical system of the heart.

When your heart suddenly starts beating too fast because of an electrical system abnormality, its rate will usually be over 120 and can even be as high as 160 to 200. This rapidity interferes with the pumping action of the heart, so that blood flow is compromised. You may experience symptoms of light-headedness or a pounding sensation in your heart. Sudden changes in your heart rhythm and a rapid or irregular pulse can be dangerous, especially if you have experienced a heart ailment such as a heart attack, heart failure, or heart enlargement from high blood pressure. Many serious types of heart rhythm disturbances occur in this setting. When this happens, see a doctor immediately. If you pass out even for a short time, it is important that you be taken to immediate emergency care.

Tip 80:

An irregular, usually rapid pulse may appear with the following symptoms: "squirrels running around in your chest," heart palpitations, fluttering, skipped beats, flopping beats, sudden spells of weakness, sudden spells of dizziness, and/or heart pounding. If your pulse suddenly begins to beat irregularly, you may be experiencing a serious heart rhythm abnormality known as atrial fibrillation. This abnormality in the heart's electrical system usually results in a pulse that is both irregular and rapid.

In atrial fibrillation abnormal electrical impulses are sent irregularly and usually rapidly throughout the heart. The two upper heart chambers (atria) suddenly stop beating regularly and go into a sort of quivering spasm. The pulse becomes chaotic and often rapid. Since the two upper heart chambers no longer squeeze blood effectively into the two lower chambers, some blood pools or stagnates in the upper chambers of the heart. Blood clots may form in these stagnant areas. When this occurs, pieces of a clot can break off and travel through blood vessels to the brain, where they lodge in a vessel and block blood flow to a part of the brain. This part of the brain is damaged, causing a stroke.

Atrial fibrillation most frequently occurs in people with heart disease, but it can also occur in people who consume large amounts of alcoholic beverages or in people with an overactive thyroid associated with shaking, tremors, exhaustion, and intolerance to heat. Atrial fibrillation sometimes occurs spontaneously in healthy people.

Treatment often includes a blood thinner to prevent blood from clotting. The doctor can convert your heart to a regular rhythm with medication or electrical shock applied to your heart. Do not ignore the general weakness and heart fluttering present when atrial fibrillation occurs. Early treatment can prevent a stroke. Seek immediate medical care.

Tip 81:

An electrical abnormality of the heart known as a prolonged Q-T syndrome can cause sudden death, especially in young athletes. The red light warning signal may include an irregular heartbeat with the following symptoms: heart palpitations, fluttering, skipped beats, flopping beats, sudden spells of weakness, sudden spells of dizziness, and/or heart pounding.

The prolonged Q-T syndrome, a serious heart rhythm problem that occurs in young people, gets its name from the EKG readout, where the distance between the Q wave and the T wave is increased. People with this condition are at risk of developing a dangerously low heart rate or a dangerously fast heart rate, requiring cardiac shock or medication. This abnormality occasionally occurs in athletes, leading to sudden death on the playing field. Even if you are young, if you feel your heartbeat skipping, it is worthwhile to be evaluated by your doctor as soon as possible, because it could be an early warning of Q-T syndrome.

Tip 82:

An irregular pulse with an excessive fluid loss from diarrhea, water pills, and/or sweating, etc. can indicate changes in the minerals of your blood, such as potassium. This can cause your pulse to become irregular, with serious health consequences. The red light warning signals may include: heart palpitations, fluttering, skipped beats, flopping beats, sudden spells of weakness, sudden spells of dizziness, heart pounding, and muscle cramps in the leg.

If you have lost an excessive amount of fluid from any cause, including sweating, water pills, or prolonged or severe diarrhea, you may lose large quantities of certain minerals such as potassium. The loss of potassium can result in abnormal electrical charges in your heart, causing dangerous irregular heartbeats, which can be life-threatening. Emergency medical therapy and monitoring by a physician is necessary. Often special intravenous fluids are needed to replace these minerals.

These heart rhythm problems can also occur with an excess of minerals in the blood, such as potassium. If you experience these heart irregularities, this is not a condition you should treat yourself.

Tip 83:

If your pulse drops below 50 beats per minute, there may be a serious impairment in your heart's pacing system that could cause your heart to stop. You can also experience dizziness or weakness.

The normal heartbeat originates from the upper chamber on the right side of the heart. If this area becomes diseased (or altered by the side effect of medication), it may stop functioning, causing a sudden slowing of the pulse. It may be so profound as to cause you to pass out, or it may occur intermittently and return to normal for a while. If this is occurring even for short periods of time, you are in danger and need to see a doctor immediately.

Tip 84:

If you listen to your heart with a stethoscope and hear a swooshing sound, it may indicate a heart murmur. You should seek medical evaluation by your doctor.

A heart murmur is a swooshing sound coming from within the heart. Heart murmurs are quite common and frequently mean nothing. For example, it may be the result of blood passing rapidly but normally through one of the four valves (doors) in the heart (see Figure 9). A large percentage of adolescents have murmurs that are not caused by disease. But a murmur may be abnormal when a damaged valve in the heart contributes to making the sound. It may also occur when blood travels through an abnormal hole in a wall that separates two heart chambers.

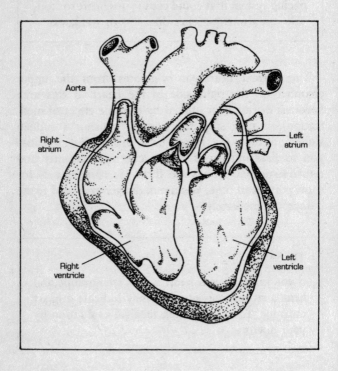

Figure 9. Inside of Heart.

To understand why blood passing through a narrowed opening makes this sound, think about a garden hose. A garden hose makes no noise when water flows from it, but if you put a nozzle on the end, a swooshing noise is created as the water spews through the narrow opening. The same thing happens with the heart, when blood flows through an abnormally narrow opening or when it flows rapidly through a normal opening. While listening to the heart with a stethoscope, the loudness, location, timing, and pitch of the murmur help the doctor to determine if the heart is damaged and where.

Certain heart murmurs must be monitored by your doctor to determine if the problem is worsening and when to correct the abnormality, to avoid permanent damage. For example, one common cause of heart murmurs is a ventricular septal defect, a birth defect where an opening in the wall of the heart separates the lower chambers. This opening causes an abnormal flow of blood, which can permanently damage the lungs. Diagnosis and treatment are essential. There are many other situations when murmurs require regular monitoring or medical intervention.

An abnormal hole in the heart, a damaged valve, a mitral valve prolapse, or an artificial valve may provide a prime target for bacterial growth (bacterial endocarditis). Therefore before undergoing any procedure on your body, it may be very important for you to take a certain antibiotic. During dental work, for example, or when tubes are put in your body to examine your bladder or colon, small amounts of bacteria can get in your blood. They may then grow on the abnormal heart valve or near the abnormal hole in your heart. But the antibiotic will kill any germs that get into your blood before they do damage.

Belly, Stomach Area, or Abdomen

How to Assess Belly Pain

1. Where, specifically, is your belly pain?

Many things can go wrong inside the belly cavity and cause pain. Some are serious and can endanger life, while others may not require any treatment. The location of the pain may provide a valuable clue as to what is wrong. Often the location of the pain points to the organ that is involved, but not always, so one clue may not be enough.

Let's divide the belly area into four sections (see Figure 10). Draw an imaginary line horizontally across the belly at the level of the belly button. Draw a second line vertically from the lower tip of the breastbone through the belly button to the pelvic bone. This effectively divides the belly into four areas or quadrants: two upper, and two lower. Pains that occur in these areas often suggest problems with the organs located there (see Figure 11). The following ailments are commonly

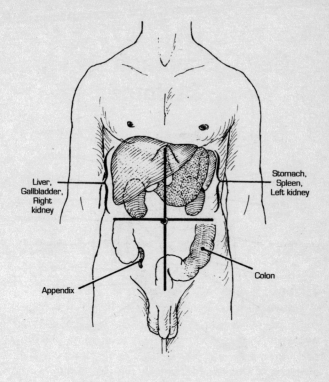

Liver,
Gallbladder,
Right
kidney

Stomach,
Spleen,
Left kidney

Colon

Appendix

Figure 10. Quadrants of the Abdomen.

located in the four quadrants (as seen from your perspective, if you were examining your own belly).

1. Your right lower quadrant: A common and poten-
    tially serious cause of pain in this area is appen-
    dicitis. Other considerations include kidney stones
    and, in women, problems with the fallopian tubes
    and ovaries.

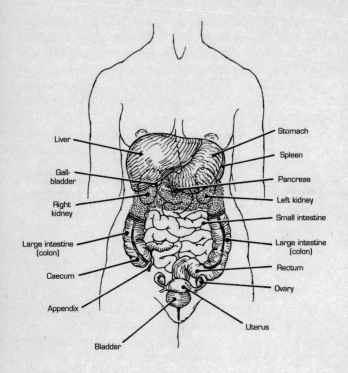

Figure 11. Evaluation of the Abdomen.

2. Your right upper quadrant: The most common cause of pain in this area is gallstones, which may lead to infection in the gallbladder. Hepatitis (liver inflammation) may also cause pain in this area.

3. Your left upper quadrant: This area contains part of the stomach, part of the colon, and the spleen. A common cause of pain in this area is gas in the colon, which is usually short-lived. Ulcers of the

stomach can cause persistent pain in this area. Injuries (e.g., from a blunt trauma to the belly) or diseases of the spleen can also cause pain here.

4. Your left lower quadrant: Pain from diverticulitis of the large bowel, kidney stones, and in women, infections in the fallopian tubes and ovaries are considerations.

5. The upper half of the belly area: Stomach or duodenal ulcers and pancreatitis pains are commonly found in this region.

6. The lower half of the belly area: Pains from bladder or prostate infections, as well as infections and tumors in the fallopian tubes, ovaries, and uterus, occur in this region.

Less common causes of bellyaches are not mentioned here.

2. Is your belly pain tender when pressed upon?

Many serious causes of bellyache are accompanied by belly tenderness. It is often important to compare where the belly is tender when you press down on the area with your fingers and where an ache is felt when you are not pressing down.

Most bellyaches from minor causes, such as a "stomach virus" or flu, usually involve very little belly tenderness. But some serious causes of bellyaches have no associated tenderness, such as kidney stones.

When belly tenderness occurs, it is usually most severe over the organ that is involved. If the inflammation or infection of the involved organ worsens and irritates the inside lining of the belly cavity, the pattern of the tenderness will change, spreading over the entire abdomen.

3. Does your belly pain get worse when you release your hand from the area where it has been pressed?

After you press your fingers down on an area of the belly, then suddenly release them, usually no pain occurs. But if this maneuver causes pain (called rebound tenderness), it usually means that the inside lining of the belly cavity is being irritated, perhaps from a specific disease that is spreading over the entire abdomen. This suggests a worsening of the problem.

4. Can you feel any lumps or pulsations in your belly?

A hard area felt in the belly may mean the presence of an abnormal growth (like a tumor) or an abscess (a pus pocket). If the hard area pulsates with the heartbeat, it may be a dilated (ballooning out) artery, which needs immediate medical attention. Firmness in the belly due to a muscle spasm of the belly wall can be mistaken for a problem originating within the belly cavity.

5. How would you describe your belly pain?

How the pain started, how it feels, and where it goes are important diagnostic considerations. It is therefore valuable for you to be able to describe these symptoms to your doctor.

What kind of pain do you have? Is it a cramping pain—that is, pain similar to the pain you feel when you get diarrhea or the urgent need to have a bowel movement? This kind of pain occurs when something contracts (squeezes) or goes into a spasm. Many of the hollow organs in the belly area—intestines, stomach, and gallbladder—have unique pain receptors called pressure receptors, meaning that anything that increases the pressure on the walls of these organs beyond a certain point will cause pain. On the other hand, these organs have no receptors that can detect cutting with a sharp object. For instance, the belly may be opened up under local anesthesia, with the individual awake, without causing pain. The bowel can also be cut under these circumstances. But if the bowel is grasped and squeezed, pain will occur. This makes sense when you consider that the danger to hollow organs is blockage, causing overexpansion and the possibility of rupture. Many diseases cause overdistention, increasing pressure on the walls of these hollow organs, and the pain is often cramping or colicky (spasmodic pain).

Other kinds of bellyaches are dull, like a toothache. They often occur when organs are infected or swollen. Sharp pain can occur in the belly when something ruptures, like a cyst, dumping blood or other liquid material inside the belly cavity.

How the pain starts can be a very important consideration in diagnosing the problem. Was the onset abrupt or sudden? A sudden onset suggests that something ruptured (in the case of a sharp pain) or spasmed (in the case of cramping pain). Gradual onset with increasing severity suggests that something inside is irritated, inflamed, or infected and is getting worse as the pain and swelling increase.

Where the pain extends is another important clue. Did it start in a certain area of the belly and remain there, or did it start in one area and spread to involve the entire belly? Pain that starts in one area and spreads suggests a progression of the problem.

A unique type of pain is a sudden sharp pain that occurs in one of the lower areas of the belly, and then hurts in the top of the left shoulder as well. This usually happens with a ruptured tubal pregnancy or a ruptured ovarian cyst, if enough blood is released and it moves along the back wall of the belly cavity up to the diaphragm (the breathing muscle separating the belly cavity from the chest). Irritation of the nerve in the diaphragm projects a pain sensation to the left shoulder. A similar pain is projected to the left shoulder from a rupture of the spleen, but in that instance the bellyache occurs in the left upper area of the belly. It rarely happens on the right side, because the liver prevents the blood from getting under the diaphragm on the right.

Pain in the belly that goes through to the back usually means something is wrong with an organ attached to the back of the belly compartment, such as the pancreas, the duodenum (first part of the small intestine), or the aorta (the big artery coming down from the heart). Gallbladder pain often radiates to the back at the right shoulder blade.

•

Indigestion

Tip 85:

Indigestion may be a sign of a heart attack. You should be especially concerned about:

1. Indigestion with exercise or exertion
2. Indigestion that does not respond to the usual medicines
3. Indigestion with a dizzy sensation
4. Indigestion with a cold sweat
5. Indigestion with numbness or pain radiating to the jaw or shoulder
6. Indigestion with pressure in the chest

Most of the time indigestion is not a serious disorder. But sometimes the feeling of indigestion can be the symptom you experience if you are having a heart attack. Often it is associated with other symptoms, as just listed although indigestion alone can be the red light warning signal of a heart attack.

Under these circumstances an immediate visit to the emergency room may save your life.

Tip 86:

If you have long-term heartburn and belching that does not respond to an antacid or ulcer medication, the condition can predispose you to ulcers, bleeding, and/or cancer of the esophagus.

The tube that carries food from your mouth to your stomach is called the esophagus. When food backs up from the stomach into the esophagus (reflux) and the esophagus becomes irritated, you can develop heartburn. Often this condition responds to an antacid or ulcer medication. When this condition is severe, it can lead to ulcers, bleeding, and/or a narrowing of the esophagus, which can predispose you to cancer in the narrowed area (this usually takes place over a number of years). Therefore, if you have heartburn for a number of weeks and it does not respond to conventional treatment, it is important to have it evaluated by your doctor.

•

Belly Pain

Tip 87:

Agonizing belly pain that worsens with any movement, accompanied by rigid belly muscles and especially in a person with a history of ulcers, is often a sign of a ruptured ulcer.

Ulcer problems have a reputation for being long-standing, with frequent bouts of belly discomfort including pain, indigestion, a feeling of fullness, nausea, and other symptoms. If you have ulcers, you may have gotten used to this discomfort by intermittently taking pills during severe bouts of pain.

This situation sets the stage for the ulcer to progress, eroding deeper and deeper into the lining of the stomach or duodenum (the first part of the small intestine, just below the stomach), until a hole is formed. When this perforation occurs, food contents are released into the belly cavity along with gas (or air). Severe internal bleeding may also occur. This rupture causes immediate, agonizing abdominal pain. One characteristic of this pain is that any movement you make worsens it. You will attempt to remain perfectly still. Also, you may experience abdominal muscle spasms. The stomach contents cause intense tissue reaction in the belly lining, resulting in a reflex belly muscle spasm with boardlike muscle rigidity: If you touch the belly area, it is not soft but is like a solid board. This condition requires immediate medical attention at an emergency room.

Tip 88:

An ulcer in the stomach or duodenum (the first part of the small intestine, just below the stomach) can cause pain in the upper-middle area of the belly with or without vomiting blood, and black tarry stools, which may wake you from sleep.

An ulcer is a sore on the lining of the stomach or duodenum. It can cause pain if it penetrates the wall or causes a spasm.

Inside the stomach the chemical hydrochloric acid and associated enzymes can change a piece of meat from solid to liquid. The stomach and duodenum contain a mucous coating that covers the lining of their walls. This coating prevents the acid and enzymes from dissolving the stomach wall itself. Various substances—including nicotine, alcohol, caffeine, aspirin, some pain medicines such as ibuprofen, (Acetaminophen does not cause ulcers.) and certain bacteria—diminish these defenses, causing ulcers to form. (Also, people with hypoparathyroidism occasionally develop ulcers. See Tip 177.) Vomiting is often associated with the irritation caused by ulcers. Early medical treatment is necessary to prevent potentially life-threatening consequences, such as bleeding and perforation. Bleeding into the duodenum may result in black tarry stools that are very sticky.

Tip 89:

Mild or severe upper-middle or left belly pain extending into the back with nausea and/or vomiting may be caused by pancreatitis. The pain is often less severe when sitting up and bending forward, while it worsens when lying flat on your back. Severe cases can cause diabetes, release dangerous chemicals into the blood, and produce internal hemorrhaging. Consumption of alcohol and foods high in fat content can cause this condition or make it much worse.

The pancreas is a narrow bandlike organ one to two inches wide, extending behind the stomach across the upper belly area for three to six inches toward the left side. It has two major functions: to produce enzymes for the small intestine to digest food, and to make insulin, which is dispatched into the bloodstream. If the pancreas gets inflamed, the release of the potent enzymes into the bloodstream or the surrounding tissues can make you very ill. They may cause internal bleeding and widespread tissue damage throughout the body. Destruction of the pancreas can cause diabetes, since the hormone insulin is necessary to drive sugar from the bloodstream into body cells. Lack of insulin production causes the hyperglycemia (high sugar levels in the blood) seen in diabetes.

The pancreas can become inflamed as a consequence of gallbladder disease. The gallbladder has a tube in common with the pancreas; if gallstones pass into this tube, they can block the outflow of the digestive chemicals from the pancreas. You can also damage your pancreas by regularly drinking alcohol. Therefore if your pancreas becomes inflamed, you should stop drinking alcohol forever. Mumps, a virus, can also cause pancreatitis. Sometimes the pancreas becomes inflamed without any identifiable cause.

The most common symptom of pancreatitis is severe belly pain in the upper-middle or upper-left areas of the belly, extending through to the back, with profound vomiting. This condition warrants emergency medical evaluation and treatment, in order to avoid serious complications. Blood studies can document damage in the pancreas.

Tip 90:

A common, often curable, cause of recurrent ulcers of the stomach and duodenum is infection of their lining by a germ called *H. pylori*. The red light warning signals are episodes of upper-middle belly pain, with or without vomiting blood, and/or black tarry stools.

For many years it was thought that stress caused ulcers. Relieve the stress, and the ulcer would heal, only to come again when the stress level was again increased. This is no longer considered to be totally correct.

The exact effect of stress on the development of ulcers has not been determined, but it is now known that a common cause of recurrent ulcers of the stomach and duodenum (the first part of the small intestine) is infection by a microscopic rod-shaped germ called

Helicobacter pylori. This discovery, in many ways, has revolutionized the treatment of ulcers. Antibiotics are now often an essential ingredient in the eradication of ulcers. The use of two or three antibiotics simultaneously controls the infection, achieves ulcer healing, and stops additional ulcers from forming.

Yet major questions arise. If an ulcer is caused by an infection, where did the infection come from, and how can you keep from getting it again? At the present time, we have no definite answers to these questions. *Helicobacter pylori* occurs worldwide and is apparently acquired from the intake of contaminated food or water. But it is not known how to detect food contamination or how to kill the germ when preparing food. It is also not known whether it can be transmitted from one person to another.

A doctor can determine if you have ulcers caused by *H. pylori* by looking into your stomach and duodenum with a gastroscope (a special tube). He or she will obtain a piece of the stomach lining (biopsy) and examine it for the *H. pylori* germs. In addition, there is a test based on breath analysis for a by-product of the infection and, more recently, a blood test for the presence of the germ.

Currently treatment for *H. pylori* is being prescribed based on the breath test or the blood test alone. Of course, if you have an ulcer with heartburn (backup of stomach acid into the esophagus), you should continue to avoid foods that cause these symptoms. Treatment is usually effective without recurrence.

Ulceration can lead to serious hemorrhage as well as rupture of the stomach or duodenum, so it is very important to be evaluated and treated for this condition as soon as possible. If you are vomiting blood or passing black tarry stools, you should be seen on an emergency basis.

Tip 91:

If you experience upper-middle belly pain (with or without vomiting blood and/or black tarry stools), you may have an ulcer or inflammation in the stomach and/or an ulcer in the duodenum. Alcohol increases the risk of developing ulcers and also prevents healing of ulcers already present. It can also make pancreatitis worse, increasing the possibility of fatal complications.

Alcohol is rapidly absorbed through the stomach lining. When this occurs, acid and enzymes pour in large volumes into the stomach, prompted by the alcohol. The presence of excessive amounts of these chemicals can lead to inflammation of the stomach, the formation of ulcers and/or cause progression of ulcers already present.

When ulcers or inflammation of the stomach and duodenum (the first part of the small intestine) are a problem, stopping the intake of alcohol is important. Drinking alcohol may relieve the belly pain momentarily, but the condition will eventually get worse, with a greater risk of internal hemorrhage or bursting of the ulcer in the abdominal cavity. Black tarry stools are a sign of ulcers bleeding into the intestines.

Belly pain associated with pancreatitis from alcohol intake is potentially life-threatening. The pancreas, located in the upper belly, produces insulin to control blood sugar and very caustic chemicals (or enzymes) to help in food digestion. When pancreatitis occurs, the substances that digest food begin to digest the pancreas itself. The caustic chemicals may also be released into the bloodstream with life-threatening consequences.

If you drink a large quantity of alcohol and suddenly develop nausea, vomiting, and severe belly pain, you are at risk of tearing the inside of your esophagus. This can cause severe bleeding and dehydration.

If you drink alcohol and have upper belly pain, seek medical care to evaluate and treat this ailment and to get advice on how to stop drinking. Belly pain with bleeding (vomiting blood or excreting black tarry stools) requires emergency medical care. (See Tip 117 for more information on black tarry stools and life-threatening bleeds.) Upper-middle and/or upper-left belly pain that extends to the back is a sign of pancreatitis and also requires emergency medical care. (See Tip 89 for more information on pancreatitis.)

Tip 92:

If you have upper-middle belly pain (with or without vomiting blood and black tarry stools), you may have an ulcer. Smoking makes stomach ulcers worse.

Smoking may cause ulcers, and it definitely retards the healing of stomach and duodenal ulcers already present. Nicotine is an active drug that has a direct, injurious effect on the lining of the stomach and duodenum. Consequently ulcers can develop and may not heal.

Stop smoking, especially if stomach and duodenal ulcers are a problem. You are at a higher risk of hemorrhage and ulcers bursting into the belly cavity. Seek medical evaluation and treatment. If you are also vomiting blood or have black tarry stools, you need emergency medical care. (See Tip 117 for more information on black tarry stools and life-threatening bleeds.)

Tip 93:

Upper-middle belly pain and/or bloody vomitus and/or black tarry stools can be caused by certain pain pills. These medicines can cause ulceration of the stomach and duodenum, which may lead to hemorrhage and bursting of the stomach in the area of the ulcer. This problem results in as many as 7,600 deaths in one year in the United States.

Aspirin, ibuprofen, Advil, Nuprin, Motril, BC Powder, Goody's, and other similar medicines (known as nonsteroidal anti-inflammatory drugs, or NSAIDs) are heavily marketed for general pain relief and the relief of joint pain in arthritis. The same medicines are prescribed by doctors in higher dosages for arthritis and other bone and muscle pains. These substances are also a major cause of ulcers and irritation of the stomach and duodenum. Ulceration caused by long-term use of these drugs can be life-threatening when it results in hemorrhaging into the stomach or duodenum. You will develop bloody vomitus (or coffee grounds in appearance) or black tarry bowel movements. Also, the ulcers can burst, causing corrosive chemicals in the stomach to leak into the belly cavity.

Take these medications only if necessary and only as directed. If you are experiencing belly pain, see your doctor immediately so that you can be evaluated and treated. There are other medications that your doctor can prescribe, along with drugs to prevent ulcer formation. If you experience belly discomfort and are vomiting blood, or if you note black tarry stools, seek emergency medical care. (See Tip 117 for more information on black tarry stools and life-threatening bleeds.)

Tip 94:

Pain in the upper-right belly area (with or without nausea and vomiting) often after eating fatty foods may be due to gallstones. If the upper-right belly becomes tender and the pain persists, and/or you develop a fever the gallbladder may be infected.

The gallbladder is located in the upper-right area of the belly, under the liver. It serves as a reservoir for bile, a substance made by the liver to help digest fat. When a fatty meal passes through the stomach and enters the first part of the small intestine (the duodenum), a hormone is released that stimulates the gallbladder to squeeze bile through the bile duct into the intestine. When bile is stored in the gallbladder, crystallized stones sometimes form. When the teardrop-shaped gallbladder contracts (squeezes), these stones may be forced into its narrow neck. As the gallbladder attempts to force the stones through its duct opening, it develops spasms, causing severe pain in the upper-right area of the belly. Nausea, vomiting, and distention in the upper-right belly area are often present as well. The pain may be constant or intermittent, and may occur more often after eating meals high in fat content.

If a gallstone is impacted in the neck of the gallbladder (like a cork in a bottle), the gallbladder balloons out, becomes infected, and sometimes ruptures.

If a gallstone passes from the gallbladder neck into the common bile duct (a tubelike structure leading from the liver to the intestine) and blocks it, yellow jaundice will occur. Your skin and/or the white part of your eye will turn yellow from the yellow bile backing up into your liver and bloodstream, spreading to all parts of your body, including your eyes. Blockage of the common bile duct can cause infection or liver failure and death.

Removal of the stone can save your life. Surgeons are able to remove the gallbladder using a fairly simple technique, inserting a special type of scope into the belly cavity.

Rarely gallstones can form in the tubes in the liver. Therefore it is possible to experience these symptoms even after your gallbladder has been removed. Medical evaluation is appropriate.

Gallstones are more commonly seen in obese women in their forties who have had several children.

If you experience upper-right belly pain often after eating fatty foods, with or without nausea and vomiting, seek medical evaluation as soon as possible. Fever indicates infection requiring immediate treatment. (See Tip 120 for more information on gallbladder disease.)

Tip 95:

Mild tenderness over the liver, swelling of the ankles and/or belly, and yellow jaundice may be signs of hepatitis and/or a scarred liver (cirrhosis). Drinking alcoholic beverages in excess and over a long period of time can cause liver disease that leads to liver cirrhosis, liver failure, and death.

Drinking any alcoholic beverage (including liquor, beer, or wine) may cause injury to the liver. When an alcoholic beverage is consumed, the alcohol is rapidly absorbed through the stomach and small intestinal wall into the bloodstream. The breakdown of alcohol occurs mainly in the liver, where certain by-products cause alcoholic hepatitis, or inflammation in liver cells. The liver cells may be destroyed and replaced with scars. The condition of a scarred liver is called cirrhosis. When enough liver cells are destroyed, liver failure and death follow.

The onset of liver cell inflammation from alcohol can be subtle, producing few symptoms. There is no severe liver pain. Instead there may be mild tenderness over the liver and occasional nausea. As the inflammation and scarring progress, swelling develops, first in the ankles and legs. Subsequently there is swelling in the belly as fluid accumulates there. Liver failure will cause yellow jaundice and dark, tea-colored urine from the backup of yellow bile, which is made in the liver. This condition is readily diagnosable by a physician in a physical examination, with a blood test that measures liver enzymes, radiological studies, and sometimes a liver biopsy.

Liver inflammation is not a disease of "drunks." You do

not have to be a heavy drinker to develop this condition. You may say, "I don't drink the hard stuff," or "I limit my drinking to beer only," but this type of liver inflammation occurs in beer drinkers as well as liquor and wine drinkers. Alcoholic hepatitis, even when severe (you turn yellow), can be reversed if alcohol intake is eliminated early enough and medical treatment is instituted. The consequence of restarting alcohol intake is often cirrhosis (scarring of the liver), causing liver failure and death. Cancer of the liver is more common in patients with cirrhosis.

Individuals with any type of non-alcohol related hepatitis are very sensitive to alcohol intake. It may increase liver inflammation and hasten the progression of liver destruction, resulting in cirrhosis.

If you have liver disease, or if you have ever had alcoholic liver disease, do not drink any alcoholic beverages. Your doctor can help you stop. Mild tenderness over the upper-right belly area, swelling of the ankles and/or belly, and/or yellow jaundice are red light warning signals that you need medical evaluation and treatment as soon as possible.

Tip 96:

An injury to the belly area can result in damage to the spleen, and a subsequent life-threatening internal hemorrhage many days after the accident. The red light warning signals may be worsening or recurring upper-left belly pain, often accompanied by left shoulder pain, and/or weakness or feeling faint. These symptoms may be felt many days after the injury.

The spleen is a spongy structure similar to a grape (but larger in size) with a soft interior, covered by a capsule. It is located in the upper-left area of the belly cavity, and it contains a large quantity of red and white blood cells. A severe blow to the belly area, from an incident such as an auto accident or a sports injury, may damage your spleen. Sudden weakness and/or fainting may indicate a life-threatening internal hemorrhage. You need to be taken to an emergency room immediately.

Sometimes, however, the injury damages the capsule of the spleen, and there is a bulging out of the internal spongy material. This condition is similar to scraping the surface of a grape and squeezing some of its contents through the damaged peel. Slowly the bulging contents may continue to come out and eventually bleed profusely. It can take many days for this to happen. Therefore you may initially experience pain, and the pain may go away and come back. Or you may develop upper-left belly pain, which persists and worsens, accompanied by left shoulder pain, due to nerve connections running on the inside of your back between the spleen and the left shoulder. Or you may suddenly become weak and faint hours or even days after the injury. It is very important to watch out for any of these symptoms after a blunt injury to the belly area. Recurring or worsening pain in the upper-left belly area, with or without left shoulder pain, deserves immediate attention at an emergency room. Sudden weakness and fainting require emergency transport to an emergency center. (See Tip 7 for more information on dizziness and life-threatening internal bleeding.)

If you have a present history of infectious mononucleosis, your spleen is more susceptible to rupture from blunt injury to your abdomen.

> **Tip 97:**
>
> If you are middle-aged or older and have sudden lower-left belly pain (sometimes, though rarely, it can occur on the right side) with intermittent constipation or diarrhea, you may have diverticulitis. If untreated, this condition can cause the colon to rupture, requiring emergency surgery.

Probably more than 30 percent of Americans have diverticulosis, a condition that usually occurs in the forties and fifties. Diverticula are small pouches formed in the cavity in the colon through which stools pass. As the colon squeezes the breakdown products of food to form stools, weakened areas of the colon wall bulge out, forming dead-end paths or diverticula. This disease may be inherited.

Diverticula can become irritated and infected (called diverticulitis) from stools or food products like seeds. Constipation can lead to infection as well. If the infected diverticula burst, the infected material can spread throughout the belly cavity, causing pus pockets, or drainage to the skin, bladder, etc., scarring, and/or blockage of the bowel, which requires emergency surgery. Diverticulitis can usually be treated with antibiotics.

This problem can begin with only one symptom of mild lower-left belly pain. You can decrease your chances of developing diverticula by eating high-fiber foods (grains, fruits, and vegetables) and drinking lots of liquids to avoid constipation.

If you develop sudden lower-left belly pain (sometimes rarely on the right side), especially with fever, seek immediate medical evaluation.

Tip 98:

Mild lower belly pain or pain during sexual intercourse may be due to an infection of the female organs by a germ called chlamydia or other germs (including the gonorrhea germ). These bacteria can cause significant damage to the fallopian tubes and lead to a life-threatening internal hemorrhage from a tubal pregnancy (ectopic pregnancy).

Germs can cause infection of the female organs. Symptoms may be few, but scarring from the infection can block the fallopian tube, through which the egg passes, causing infertility. Also, the scarring can interfere with the small fingerlike projections located at the end of the fallopian tubes, which pick up the egg when it bursts from the ovary each month. This also leads to infertility.

Fertilization normally occurs when an egg travels along the fallopian tube to its midportion and meets with sperm. After fertilization, the egg has approximately three days to travel through the rest of the tube into the cavity of the womb, where it grows on the wall and gets nourishment from the mother's body. If this trip is delayed by scarring from infections, the fertilized egg will attach in the wall of the tube and begin to grow there. Growth of the embryo can proceed only to a limited size (usually six to eight weeks from the beginning of pregnancy) before the tube ruptures, with the potential of a life-threatening hemorrhage. Lower belly pain, weakness, dizziness, and a rapid pulse may indicate that this rupture has occurred. It requires emergency surgery.

It is important to know when your female organs are

infected, in order to prevent damage to your tubes, ovaries, and uterus. Mild discomfort in the lower belly or pain during sexual intercourse may be a clue. The presence of infection can usually be detected by testing at the mouth of the womb. Regular checkups with your doctor provide an opportunity for early detection. If you think you have had sexual contact with someone infected with chlamydia, or gonorrhea, or if you have any of these vague symptoms, tell your doctor.

Tip 99:

Red light warning signals of a serious infection called toxic shock syndrome are lower-belly pain and a high fever, often with a bright red rash all over the body. Any severe vaginal infection (sometimes associated with the use of tampons) may lead to this ailment.

Toxic shock syndrome, first observed in young menstruating women, is rare but potentially fatal. The onset of the infection is sudden and rapidly progresses from high fever and diarrhea with lower belly pain to a dramatic drop in blood pressure and death.

This disease is more common in women who put tampons in their vagina, especially for longer than normal periods of time. This may contribute to the development of an infection. It is caused by a rare strain of commonly occurring bacteria. Severe vaginal infections may be a clue that this ailment is present.

It is recommended that tampons be changed every

four to eight hours and not be used continuously throughout the menstrual cycle.

If treatment with antibiotics begins early, you can fully recover. If you have a high fever, lower belly pain, and a vaginal infection, you should see your physician as soon as possible.

Tip 100:

The red light warning signals of lower belly pain with low back pain and problems with urination, such as slowing of urine flow and/or pain on urination, indicate many different possible ailments in men. Infections of the urinary tract are important to recognize early since they can cause serious kidney disease if not treated (see Tip 122). These symptoms can also be a sign of prostatitis or prostate cancer.

If you have an infected prostate gland (prostatitis), you may experience long-term pain and tenderness in the lower belly, lower back pain, or pain in the area in back of your scrotum. You may also experience a burning sensation when you urinate and a slowing of urine flow. When the prostate swells, it causes these symptoms by pushing against the urethra (the tube leading from the bladder through the penis to the outside). On the other hand, prostatitis may also appear with a sudden high fever and aching all over your body.

The prostate may be felt during a rectal exam; therefore, a diagnosis of prostatitis can be readily made. Antibiotics are the usual treatment.

A person with advanced prostate cancer may have

symptoms of hesitancy on starting urination, slowing of urine flow, and dribbling after completing urination. The most common cause of these symptoms is a benign (noncancerous) growth of the prostate gland. Prostate cancer is much more common in men over 60 years of age, but it can also occur in younger men. The problem is that it usually causes few symptoms in the early stages and often becomes advanced before it is detected. In general, when you are old and get prostate cancer, it will act old as well. It is usually less aggressive and less likely to spread and become fatal. A blood test, the PSA, helps in the early detection of prostate cancer. The American Cancer Society recommends that men over the age of 50 receive a PSA test annually.

If you are a man with lower belly pains and/or low back pain, or urination problems, see your doctor as soon as possible for evaluation and treatment.

Tip 101:

Lower-right belly pain and tenderness may indicate appendicitis. Appendicitis is a serious disease that can be fatal if the appendix ruptures.

Typically an early diagnosis of appendicitis results in a cure with surgery. But without proper treatment, the appendix can rupture and cause infection to spread throughout the belly cavity—and this can be fatal.

Appendicitis is an inflammation of the appendix, a finger-shaped structure projecting from the first part of the colon. Swelling and inflammation at the spot where it is attached to the colon can block its blood supply, leading to gangrene in its tip and rupture.

Appendicitis often causes a bellyache. Initially this pain may be vague and spread throughout the belly. Eventually the pain will often (but not always) localize to the lower-right area of the belly, which will be tender to the touch. This usually occurs over a forty-eight-hour period and will continue to get worse until the appendix ruptures, at which time the pain lessens. So reduction of the pain may mean that you are worse, not better.

Other tip-offs that may accompany appendicitis include a low-grade fever not usually over 101.5 degrees, loss of appetite, nausea, vomiting, diarrhea, and constipation.

On occasion, the pain of appendicitis is located in other areas: the right side of the lower back (if the appendix projects up the back side of the colon) or the upper-right belly (if the first part of the colon is displaced to this area, as during pregnancy).

If you suspect appendicitis, you should go to an emergency room for immediate medical evaluation.

•

Bulges and Swelling in the Belly

Tip 102:

If you have a pulsating bulge in your belly, it may mean that the aorta, the main vessel coming out of your heart, is ballooning out (aortic aneurysm). This is life-threatening if it bursts.

The aorta, the large artery that leaves the heart, is the main passageway of blood to the rest of the body. It arches in the chest to follow the spinal column into the belly area, where it branches to both legs. If the wall of this blood vessel develops a weak spot, it can bulge out, much like the weak spots on an inner tube. The bulge is called an aneurysm. The danger is rupture of the bulge, causing sudden death from massive hemorrhage.

Symptoms of an aortic aneurysm may be vague belly pain or back pain. It may become obvious by the appearance of a pulsating mass palpable in the belly. The likelihood that an aneurysm will rupture increases as it gets larger. When it reaches a certain size, it is important to get it repaired before it bursts.

Obviously this condition needs to be diagnosed before rupture. Therefore if you note a pulsating bulge, you should let your doctor know. Occasionally an aneurysm is detected during a routine physical exam. It also may be discovered during a routine abdominal X-ray. Aneurysms are most often seen in people with high blood pressure, diabetes, and diseases where fatty deposits build up in the arterial wall; smokers; and in those with a family history of aneurysms (e.g., Marfan's syndrome). If you have an aneurysm and you suffer sudden, severe back pain and/or blood in your stools or a change in the color of your legs, with or without sweating or weakness, you need immediate transport to emergency medical care.

•

Sense of Fullness

Tip 103:

If you have had ulcers, you feel full after eating small amounts of food, and vomit frequently, you may have a blockage from scarring or growths in the stomach or duodenum (see Figure 12).

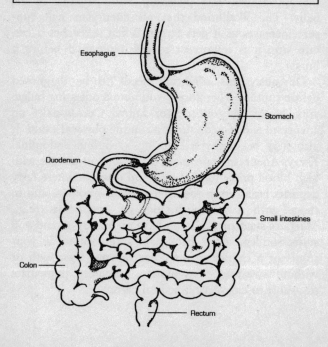

Figure 12. Intestines.

When ulcers of the stomach and duodenum (the beginning segment of the small intestine) heal, they are replaced by scar tissue. Scar tissue may shrink or contract, which results in strangling parts of the stomach or duodenum. Multiple ulcers produce multiple scars, sometimes causing blockage of the stomach or duodenum. This is an emergency.

During surgery the narrowed areas in the stomach or duodenum are opened and the scars are removed. Various segments of the intestines may need to be sewn together to bypass the blocked areas.

If you are feeling full, vomiting after small meals, and have a history of ulcers, see your doctor for medical evaluation and therapy as soon as possible.

•

Genitalia

Male

Tip 104-A:

A lump in your testicle with or without a small lump in the groin could be serious.

Tip 104-B:

Testicular cancer is more commonly found in testicles that did not naturally descend from the abdomen to the scrotum. No testicle is felt in the scrotum unless it was surgically put there.

If you notice a nonpainful, hard lump or swelling in your testicle, you need to see your physician for evaluation for testicular cancer as soon as possible.

Testicular cancer is the cancer most common in young men. The average age is 32.

Normally, as a child, your testicles descend from

your abdomen to your scrotum. If this does not happen, you are at a higher risk for developing testicular cancer. Therefore if you do not feel testicles in your scrotum, or if your testicles were surgically taken from your abdomen and placed in your scrotum, you are at a higher risk for cancer and should let your doctor know so he or she can monitor you closely.

Self-examination of your testicles for lumps once or twice a month can result in early detection of cancer. Discovering testicular cancer at an early stage and treating it can save your life. Cure rates can be as high as 90 percent, depending on the type of cancer. (See Appendix B for instructions on self-examination.)

Tip 105:

Irritation, redness, or tenderness occurring in the foreskin of the penis may be a sign of diabetes.

Blood testing to diagnose diabetes is important in men with infections in the foreskin of the penis. Early therapy can decrease the complications of diabetes, including eye, heart, and kidney problems.

•

Male and Female

Tip 106:

A nonpainful, raw-looking sore located on or near the penis, vaginal area, or breast or mouth can be an early sign of syphilis.

This type of sore may be an early warning sign of a disease that can be fatal. Initially syphilis begins as an ugly-looking sore with a hard rim around it. It heals on its own.

During the next stage of the disease, you may notice a rash on your body (see Tip 142). It too disappears on its own. The final phase of syphilis is when the infecting germ damages one of the valves (doors) in your heart and/or destroys brain cells, causing mental deterioration. Syphilis is curable if you receive antibiotics when you first notice the sore with the hard rim around it. Therefore if you have a non-painful, raw-looking sore near the genitals and/or mouth, see your doctor as soon as possible.

•

Female

Tip 107:

An early sign of a potentially serious infection of the female organs is a foul-smelling, thick, greenish discharge from the vagina often with lower-belly discomfort.

A discharge like the one just described is often the first sign of a serious infection in the female organs. Irritation of the vagina may be the only other symptom. The infection can spread into your womb (uterus), fallopian tubes, and belly cavity. This condition is called pelvic inflammatory disease (PID), which causes severe lower belly pain that is tender to the touch. You may have a fever of 101 degrees or higher, with weakness, nausea, vomiting, and generalized aching. Pelvic pus pockets can form, and the infection can spread throughout the body. Scarring may occur in the area around the womb, which can impair fertility or even cause sterility. The scarring increases the risk of having a pregnancy in the fallopian tubes, which can burst, causing life-threatening internal hemorrhage. (See Tip 181.)

Early medical evaluation and treatment of the discharge (especially with lower belly discomfort) can prevent the dangerous spread of the infection.

Tip 108:

Yeast infections cause a red sore on the skin with a buttermilk or cottage-cheese-type discharge from the vagina, or a white patch. Repeated yeast infections in the vagina, on the skin, or in the corners of the mouth may be a warning sign of diabetes or AIDS.

Yeast infections of the vagina frequently occur after a woman takes an antibiotic, because the antibiotic kills the normal bacteria in the vagina, allowing the ever-present yeast to overgrow. Often a white clumpy discharge (like cottage cheese) will occur. These infections usually clear promptly after treatment with an antifungal medication.

Other common sites for yeast infections are on the skin near the groin, under the breasts, in the corners of the mouth, and even inside the mouth. They are often accompanied by a burning sensation and a white discharge or plaque. Often these infections are responsive to antifungal medication.

If you have repeated yeast infections, you should be tested for diabetes. High sugar levels in the blood·and a defective defense system against infection increase the incidence of these yeast infections. Early diagnosis of diabetes with proper therapy can reduce your risk of serious complications, including kidney, blood vessel, and heart damage.

HIV infection can also cause repeated yeast infections, because the natural body defenses (the immune system) are weakened. Testing for HIV is appropriate for early treatment and preventive measures to limit the spread of the disease to others.

Tip 109:

A wart in the genital area in women may be a warning sign for the risk of developing cancer of the cervix (mouth of the womb).

A small, moist fingerlike projection in the genital area may be caused by the human papilloma virus. The presence of the human papilloma virus increases the risk of developing cancer of the cervix. It is important to see a physician for a thorough pelvic examination on a regular basis for early detection in case cancer changes occur. The Pap smear is the test used to check for abnormalities of the cervix, and it should be performed once a year.

Tip 110:

If you are an older woman (after menopause) and you are experiencing redness, itching, white patches, and/or an ulcer that does not heal in or near your genitals, you may have cancer. Cancer in this region may appear not as a growth but as an irritated or ulcerated area.

Thinning of the skin in the genital area occurs as a result of a decrease in the levels of the hormone estrogen and as part of the aging process. Cancer of the lips of the vulva (the outside of the vagina) usually occurs long after menopause. It is a type of skin cancer, but it may appear only as an irritated area and may or may not have an ulceration. These red light warning signals need to be evaluated by your doctor as soon as possible. They may go unnoticed unless you see your doctor on a regular basis for checkups.

•

Bowel Movement

Pain

Tip 111:

Anal pain that does not immediately improve with common hemorrhoid treatment needs medical attention. You could have a life-threatening abscess (pus pocket) around the rectum.

The anal area is very sensitive and can get quite painful when irritated. When severe pain occurs in this area, you will probably assume you have hemorrhoids. Most likely you will follow the basic treatment of hot baths, foods or medications that soften your stools, and suppositories and wait for the symptoms to go away. If the pain is actually caused by hemorrhoids, they will probably clear up with this treatment. But if you have formed a pus pocket (perirectal abscess), the waiting could be costly.

This pus pocket is formed when germs gain entrance to the anal wall and set up an infection. The infection spreads through the anal wall into an open space between muscles in the buttocks area. This empty space is similar to the space, in the wall of a house, between the sheetrock and the outside wall. In this location the infection will not show up like a boil or abscess and will not come to a head. The germs spread farther upward along the wall of the rectum. The pain caused by these abscesses increases steadily. Surgery is the only treatment to stop the spreading infection. During surgery the pus pocket is cut open and drained.

When you suffer from rectal pain, remember that it may not be from hemorrhoids. Do not allow the pain to persist too long before getting it checked by a physician.

•

Form and Frequency

Tip 112:

If you develop a change in your bowel habits (excluding a short episode of diarrhea) or begin to pass pencil-size slivers of stools, then you need to be evaluated. It could be an early sign of cancer of the colon. Also, other diseases affecting the intestines can cause these red light warning signals.

The pattern of bowel movement frequency is an individual trait. Some people have a bowel movement every day, while others have one every other day or every third day. Any of these patterns can be normal for you and is no cause for alarm.

An important red light warning signal is when the pattern of bowel movement suddenly changes. This is true whether your bowel movements become more frequent or less frequent. It means that something is disturbing the normal function of the colon, and that something could be cancer.

Another red light warning signal is a change in the diameter of the bowel movement. Usually the diameter of the formed stool that is passed reflects the diameter of the colon. A narrowing of the colon brought on by a constricting growth such as cancer may cause the stool to become consistently narrow in diameter with the appearance of a pencil.

Since early evaluation increases the chance of a cure for colon cancer or detecting other diseases of the intestines, being sensitive to such minor changes in the body's function may save your life. When they occur, see your doctor.

Tip 113:

A bout of severe diarrhea or diarrhea lasting more than forty-eight hours can be fatal.

A sudden and severe infectious diarrhea can be caused by many different bacteria (*Campylobacter, Salmonella, Shigella*) or by other germs called protozoans (*Entamoeba, Giardia,* and *Cryptosporidia*). They can make you sick with profuse, bloody, life-threatening diarrhea. Severe diarrhea or diarrhea that lasts longer than forty-eight hours can cause such severe dehydration (fluid loss) and loss of essential minerals that intravenous fluids and replacement of minerals are necessary on an emergency basis.

One of the most severe types of life-threatening diarrhea is called pseudomembranous colitis. It is caused by a toxin from a bacterium called *Clostridium difficile.* The diarrhea is often thick with blood and mucus and may look as though you are shedding the lining of your colon. It can result in dehydration accompanied by extreme toxicity, which can be fatal. If you are taking an antibiotic for an infection someplace else in your body, it can kill the normal bacteria that live in your colon and promote growth of the rare bacterium that causes pseudomembranous colitis.

Another bacterium that causes diarrhea, often among a number of people at once, is *E. coli.* Epidemics caused by *E. coli* result from eating undercooked beef or by ingesting water that has been contaminated (as in a swimming pool).

One of the most dangerous and infectious types of diarrhea is cholera. It is rare in the Western world but is common in developing countries. Before traveling abroad, check with your local health department to get the appropriate preventive therapy. In addition to germs, many other illnesses also cause diarrhea.

In all cases of diarrhea you can become dehydrated (feeling dizzy, weak, etc.) and lose essential minerals, such as potassium. Therefore it is always important to replenish fluids and minerals and determine the underlying cause of the diarrhea. Do not allow diarrhea to persist without contacting your doctor. Diarrhea containing blood causing weight loss, associated with fever, or which awakens you at night, needs to be assessed by a physician as soon as possible.

Tip 114:

Bowel movements that occur less often than every three days usually mean you are constipated. Constipation can be a sign of various diseases of the colon, including cancer. Early diagnosis and treatment can prevent serious complications.

After digestion is completed in the stomach and small intestine, food residues arrive in the colon. The colon is a muscular walled tube five to six feet in length. It conserves body water by removing 90 percent of the water from the food residues (fecal material) as they pass through. If the transit time in the colon is too slow, too much water is removed, and the feces become hard, which causes constipation. If the transit time is too fast, the fecal material will come out as diarrhea.

Constipation is often caused by weak muscles in the wall of the colon. Some individuals inherit this trait, while others weaken the muscles of the colon wall by using laxatives too frequently. You can actually become dependent on laxatives. Many medications, including certain ones for pain and blood pressure and those containing iron, can cause constipation. Numerous diseases of the colon, including cancer, cause constipation, which needs to be ruled out by a doctor. Early treatment of the underlying illness often can prevent serious complications. Other ailments, including hypothyroidism (low thyroid gland function), can also cause constipation.

Measures to relieve constipation are directed at improving the colon's ability to propel material through it. Increased water consumption helps prevent the fecal material from becoming too hard. Stool softeners also help. Some laxatives stimulate the colon wall to squeeze fecal material through more easily, while others irritate the bowel lining, which prompts the flow of water back into the colon to aid the flow of fecal material. The latter type of laxative is less desirable because it further weakens the bowel wall. The dietary fiber present in vegetables, grain, and fruits and in powder supplements are important ways to facilitate the movement of feces through the colon. Also increased water intake and exercise are often helpful.

If you have a bowel movement less often than every three days, see your doctor for an evaluation to determine the underlying cause.

Tip 115:

Cramping belly pain with a swollen belly, vomiting, and no passage of gas or bowel movement for more than twenty-four hours may mean life-threatening bowel blockage.

An unrelieved intestinal blockage is fatal. It may take many days or weeks before you get very sick. The pain and vomiting will most likely compel you to seek medical care before the condition becomes life-threatening.

The bowel can be blocked either in the small intestine

or in the large intestine. When blocked, fecal material and gas back up. As the bowel attempts to force material through the blockage, you experience severe cramping belly pain. If the location of the blockage is high up in the small bowel, vomiting will occur early on. If the blockage is low in the colon, vomiting will occur late or not at all.

Prior abdominal surgery is the most common cause of bowel obstruction. Scar tissue or adhesions occur after such surgery. Often these adhesions are "bandlike," stretching from one organ to another. These "bands" may cause entrapment of a loop of bowel, kinking it sufficiently to block it. The intestine is a tubular garden-hose-type structure. It becomes kinked when it gets entangled in these bands of scar tissue, which block the flow of contents through the intestines. When left untreated, the entanglement may cut off the blood circulation to the bowel wall, causing gangrene of the loop of bowel that is entrapped. If the blockage is not relieved by surgery, death can occur.

Cancerous growths or severe inflammation and infection of the colon can cause colon blockage. It can also occur from thick, solid, hard stools accumulating in the rectum (an impaction). Treatment of an impaction includes enemas. If the treatment is not successful, the blockage can often be removed by a health professional sticking a gloved finger up the rectum and carefully removing the hardened stools. This condition is more common in senior citizens or dehydrated bedridden patients.

If you are nauseated, vomiting, or experiencing lower belly pain with swelling and have not passed gas or a bowel movement in twenty-four hours, you should seek immediate medical attention.

•
Color

Tip 116:

**Anytime dark or bright red blood appears in the
bowel movement, an early medical evaluation
and treatment may save your life.**

There are many reasons that you may pass blood from
the rectum. Bright red blood that appears on toilet tissue
could be a sign of colon cancer; removing it early could
save your life. The thought that "It's only hemorrhoids"
has put a lot of colon cancer victims in early graves.
Remember, even if you have hemorrhoids, the rectal bleeding could also be from cancer. Rectal bleeding should be
considered a sign of cancer until proven otherwise.

Blood from the rectum can originate from anywhere
in the gastrointestinal (GI) tract, from the mouth all the
way to the anus. Possible sources of bleeding are irritation and ulcers in the mouth, stomach, or intestines, as
well as cancer in these areas. Even swallowing blood
from a nosebleed can cause blood to appear in your
bowel movements. Usually the darker the blood, the
higher up the bleeding site in the GI tract. The stools can
become black and tarry. A thorough examination
includes special X-rays or passing an endoscope (a special tube with a miniature video camera) into the mouth
to examine the esophagus, stomach, and upper small
intestine. A sigmoidoscope (another tube with a minia-

ture video camera) is passed into the anus to examine sections of the large intestine. A colonoscope can reach all of the large intestine (colon). These procedures are not as uncomfortable as they might seem.

Sometimes the earliest sign of bleeding in the GI tract is a low blood count (anemia). A very sensitive test, placing fecal material on a special card, can detect blood in the stool that is not seen on visual inspection. This can be a tip-off to an early stage of cancer, when your only abnormality is a low blood count.

Cancer of the colon is one of the more common cancers. If you have a close relative who has had colon cancer, you are at greater risk. If you have a family history of colon polyps, you should establish a program of routine colonoscopy, even if you are young and do not have any symptoms. Whether you have a family history or not, routine screening sigmoidoscopy every five years and checking for microscopic amounts of blood in the stool every year may be lifesaving. The American Cancer Society recommends that colon cancer screening begin at age 50.

Early detection without any warning signs can lead to a cure of the cancer. This disease is not rare!

Also, remember, if you pass red or dark blood in your bowel movement, seek medical evaluation as soon as possible.

Tip 117:

Black tarry stools may indicate a hemorrhage from an ulcer of the stomach or duodenum. It is important to stop the bleeding and to rule out cancer as a cause.

When an ulcer in the stomach or duodenum (the first part of the small intestine) erodes into a blood vessel, hemorrhage will occur. If the vessel is small, the blood loss may be only a trickle, but if the vessel is large, bleeding will be brisk and life-threatening.

Bleeding a little from small vessels in the stomach or duodenum may go unnoticed. The blood can be spread out through the twenty feet of small bowels and five to six feet of large bowel (the colon). This bleeding can be detected by placing a small amount of stool on a test card, which will change color if blood is present.

Blood originating from the stomach or duodenum often turns pitch black from chemicals (enzymes) in the small bowel. The stools can also take on a tarry consistency, especially if the bleeding is rapid. Belly pain caused by an ulcer may lessen when bleeding occurs because blood at the ulcer site coats the sore and protects it from the acid of the stomach. Nausea and vomiting are often not present unless there is a rapid flow of blood in the stomach. In this case the vomiting may increase in frequency and volume.

There are other red light warning signals of blood loss. You may become very weak from a low blood count (anemia). If the loss of blood volume is severe, standing up may make you feel weak and light-headed. The blood pressure drops and the pulse rises. Under these circumstances death can occur rapidly unless emergency treatment is instituted.

Suppose you have just vomited blood. It occurred only once, and you otherwise feel pretty good. But you notice that your pulse is 100 beats per minute. Do not ignore the presence of a fast pulse—take immediate action. The pulse is the most sensitive measure of rapid blood loss. If the pulse is above 90, or higher

than your normal pulse, emergency medical assistance
is needed.

The safest approach is to always seek immediate medical evaluation and treatment when you first note that
you are passing black tarry stools.

Tip 118:

**The passage of pale, putty-colored stools can be
due to blockage of substances normally secreted
by the liver into the intestine.**

Stools are normally dark or light brown or green in
color. If the stool loses its color, becoming a pale clay or
putty color, it means that there is a lack of pigment passing from the liver into the intestines. This indicates a
blockage of the bile duct that carries these substances
from the liver into the intestines. It often indicates that
you have liver disease, or that a gallstone or tumor is
blocking the bile duct.

You should report this finding to your doctor as soon
as possible, so that appropriate evaluation and treatment can be instituted. There is a potential for developing serious complications including permanent liver
damage.

Urine

Appearance

Tip 119:

Blood in the urine without pain can be more serious than when there is pain.

The most common causes of blood in the urine—kidney stones and a bladder or prostate infection—are usually accompanied by many symptoms. The agonizing pain of kidney stones or the burning discomfort and urinary frequency of a bladder or prostate infection gets people to the doctor early. But when blood appears in your urine without accompanying pain, especially in a single episode, you may take a "wait and see" attitude. This attitude may have dire consequences.

If you see blood in the urine, tell your doctor as soon

as possible. There are many causes of bleeding into the urinary tract, and one of them is cancer, which may be in the kidney, the ureter, the bladder, or the prostate. At the time when they are still curable, these cancers often do not cause pain. Therefore blood in the urine may be the only clue for an early diagnosis.

Among the other causes of blood in the urine are infections, stones, kidney disease, and exercise, even when all structures are normal.

Tip 120:

Tea-colored urine and/or yellow skin or eyes, with or without nausea and a sense of fullness, may indicate repeated problems with gallstones. If untreated, this condition can cause liver failure, pancreatitis, or bursting of the gallbladder. Other causes of these symptoms can be damaged red blood cells and any liver ailments including hepatitis and cancer.

It is natural for urine to darken in color, especially in hot weather, when the body loses fluid through sweat and the urine becomes concentrated. But the dark color of this urine is nowhere close to the tea-colored urine that occurs when excess bilirubin appears in the urine. Bilirubin is normally processed in the liver and turned into bile. Bile is stored in the gallbladder and flows in a tube (the bile duct) to the intestines to help digest fat.

If gallstones form in the gallbladder and gain entrance to the bile duct, they often block the flow of bile to the intestines. The bile will then back up into the liver, causing inflammation. This results in a feeling of nausea and a sense of fullness. The backup of bile may result in an accumulation of bilirubin in the blood. This yellow substance turns your skin and eyes yellow and your urine a tea color. When the gallstone passes through the bile duct into the intestine, the urine clears. But if another stone from the gallbladder gets stuck in the bile duct, these signs and symptoms are repeated. If this continues to occur, it can permanently damage the liver. Also, the blockage of the bile duct can cause the gallbladder to swell and rupture, resulting in toxic substances flowing into the belly cavity.

Another complication of gallstones can occur if a stone passes from the bile duct to a duct that is also connected to the pancreas. This tube carries very caustic digestive substances from the pancreas to the small intestines. A backup of these substances can be fatal, leading to inflammation of the pancreas (pancreatitis).

It should be noted that liver ailments, including hepatitis and cancer of the liver, can also cause an excess of bilirubin in the blood, causing tea-colored urine and yellow skin and eyes. Also, red blood cells in the bloodstream are a source of bilirubin. Any disease or side effect of a drug that breaks up red blood cells can cause bilirubin to accumulate in the blood.

If your urine turns tea-colored, or if your skin or eyes turn yellow, it is imperative that you seek medical attention.

Tip 121:

A rare abnormal opening between the bladder and colon can cause you to pass bubbles while you urinate. It can lead to severe infections. This condition can be caused by scarring or cancer.

Scarring or cancer can cause connections (fistulas) between the bowel and the bladder. An early sign may be passing bubbles while you urinate. The bubbles are caused by gas in the bowels passing into the bladder. The urine will eventually become foul-smelling, with debris from the colon. Seek evaluation and treatment by a urologist (surgical kidney and bladder specialist) as soon as possible.

•

Discomfort

> **Tip 122:**
>
> Discomfort during urination—usually burning—a recurrent feeling that you need to urinate, and/or the need to urinate frequently are symptoms of a bladder infection. Repeated urinary tract infections may indicate a blockage in the plumbing system of your body and may cause kidney failure.

Bladder infections cause spasms resulting in frequent urination, a recurrent feeling that you need to urinate, and/or burning discomfort on urination. These infections are common and treatable with antibiotics.

Women are more likely to have urinary tract infections, due to the shortness of the urethra (the tube from the bladder to the outside). A germ can get into the bladder more easily.

If a man has more than one urinary tract infection or if

a woman has more than two, it may be a tip-off of an abnormality. The abnormality may be in the tube that carries urine from the kidney to the bladder (ureter), in the bladder itself, or in the tube from the bladder to the outside of your body (urethra). It impedes the free flow of urine.

A bladder infection that does not respond to antibiotic therapy is another red light warning signal indicating these problems. Anything that blocks, delays, or reverses the flow of urine can lead to a urinary tract infection that will recur unless the altered flow pattern is corrected. Examples of such defects include:

1. Kidney stones in the kidney or in the ureter (the tube that goes from the kidney to the bladder)
2. A kink in the ureter
3. A growth in any adjacent organ pressing on the ureter
4. Vesico-ureteral reflux, a condition that allows urine to reverse its flow from the bladder back up into the ureter
5. An anatomical veil in the urethra that partially blocks the urine flow from the bladder
6. Urethral stricture, or narrowing of the urethra

If not corrected, these problems may cause recurrent kidney infections, resulting in kidney failure, the need to be routinely connected to a kidney machine (dialysis), or a kidney transplant.

Other causes of repeated urinary tract infections include disorders of the immune system and diabetes, which also require treatment.

If you experience a painful burning or frequent urination, you should see a doctor as soon as possible. Repeated bladder infections or poor response to therapy indicate that you need a thorough evaluation by a urologist (surgical kidney specialist).

•

Frequency

Tip 123:

If you are having difficulty passing urine or cannot urinate at all, you need urgent relief. It is very important to determine the cause, which can be lifesaving. Permanent correction is necessary to avoid kidney failure.

The inability to urinate requires urgent relief. If you are not able to urinate, try sitting in a tub of warm water three to four inches deep. After a few minutes, try to urinate in the water. Your discomfort can be relieved by being catheterized (having a tube placed into the bladder, usually by a doctor or a nurse).

In situations when you can only partially empty your bladder, urine remains and accumulates there—a prime setup for infection. If untreated, such an infection can spread into the kidneys and destroy them.

What causes this problem? In men, an enlarged prostate gland may be blocking the flow of urine from the bladder since the tube to the outside runs through the prostate. In women and men, the urethra, the tube from the bladder to the outside of the body, may be narrowed. An infection can irritate and scar this tube so that urine cannot pass through. Another cause is a loss of strength in the muscles in the wall of the bladder, such that they are no longer strong enough to force urine through the narrowed outflow passage. Diabetes or multiple sclerosis can damage the nerves responsible for squeezing the bladder. Antihistamines and other over-the-counter medicines can constrict or partially close the bladder opening. The longer the inability to urinate exists, the more the bladder wall expands, making it thinner and weaker. This weakened wall is less able to squeeze urine out of the bladder. It becomes difficult to urinate.

If the passageway from the bladder to the outside of the body is blocked, effective treatment may include medication or a procedure to permanently unblock it. In men with a large prostate, a PSA blood test, an ultrasound, and/or a biopsy of the prostate tissue will help to determine if the enlargement is due to cancer. Early detection and treatment of cancer can be lifesaving.

In conclusion, when you have difficulty urinating, see your doctor immediately or go to an emergency room for urgent relief. You need timely follow-up by a urologist (surgical kidney specialist) to evaluate and treat the underlying problem.

Tip 124:

Weight loss, increased urination, blurred distance vision, and increased thirst and appetite are highly suggestive of diabetes. The early stages of diabetes often have no symptoms, and the only way to know if you have it is to have your blood sugar checked.

Weight loss is a sign of many disorders. But when you have an increased appetite and are continuously thirsty along with significant weight loss, you may have a certain type of diabetes. This condition also causes frequent urination. Type 1 diabetes occurs when cells in the pancreas stop secreting insulin, the hormone responsible for transporting sugar in the blood to your body cells.

When the sugar increases in the blood, it will pass into the urine. This pulls extra fluid into the urine, causing increased urination. Distance vision may also be blurred. Therefore you drink more to replenish your fluids and continue urinating a lot. The loss of sugar in your urine results in losing calories and hence weight. Due to the lack of insulin, the body cannot use the sugar as a source of energy.

Diabetes can be diagnosed by obtaining a fasting blood sugar test, which means you do not eat for at least eight hours before the test. A fasting blood sugar level of 126 mg/dl or higher suggests the diagnosis of diabetes.

If you have diabetes, it is important to keep track of your blood sugar levels. You can use a glucometer with a test strip (available at pharmacies) to check the sugar in your blood. Also, your doctor can obtain a very helpful blood test, called hemoglobin A1c, to get an average assessment of your blood sugar level over a period of three months. This test is particularly valuable because the complications of diabetes are closely related to the long-term continuous control of blood sugar levels.

Diagnosing this disease early is important so that treatment can be instituted to prevent complications. These include kidney disease, blindness, heart ailments, skin problems, and damage to blood vessels. Diabetes may lead to the loss of toes, feet, or legs as a result of the buildup of fat deposits in the blood vessels, which blocks the supply of nourishment and oxygen to these specific areas of the body.

Type 1 diabetes is treated with insulin injections. A balanced diet with limited carbohydrates and minimal sugar intake is recommended. In addition, a healthy exercise program tailored to your needs is advisable.

On the other hand, Type 2 diabetes is caused by a combination of insufficient insulin plus resistance to the action of insulin. Weight loss and exercise improve insulin action and are helpful. A special diet is also important, and sometimes medications are needed to control blood sugar levels.

If you experience increased urination, appetite, and thirst, often with weight loss, seek medical evaluation to determine if you have diabetes or there is another cause for these symptoms.

•

Menstruation (Periods), Menopause, and PMS

Irregular Periods

> **Tip 125:**
>
> Too much bleeding at the time of your period, an abnormally long period, or bleeding off and on between periods can be a sign of a serious disease.

Normally your body's menstrual periods occur every twenty-eight days, give or take seven days, and last approximately four days. If your periods occur fewer than twenty-one days apart, if they last more than seven days, or if you experience intermittent bleeding, then you have an abnormal bleeding pattern.

Abnormal vaginal bleeding can be an indication of cancer of the uterus (womb). Early diagnosis provides an opportunity for treatment and cure for the two types of uterine cancer: (1) cancer of the cervix (mouth of the womb), and (2) cancer of the endometrium (lining of the womb). Both of these types of cancer can produce abnormal vaginal bleeding. Remember, abnormal vaginal bleeding does not have to be heavy to indicate cancer. Even a small amount of bleeding between normal periods or after intercourse can be significant: The American Cancer Society recommends that women begin yearly pap smears at the age of 18 or when they become sexually active, whichever comes first. Pap smears can detect cancer of the cervix early, even before abnormal bleeding occurs.

Pap smears do not detect cancer of the lining of the womb. The appearance of abnormal vaginal bleeding is usually the only clue that this cancer is present.

An overgrowth of the lining of the womb, though noncancerous, is another cause of excessive and prolonged vaginal bleeding. This condition, usually a result of hormone problems, causes irregular shedding of the lining of the womb and thus abnormal, often heavy menses. This condition may be precancerous.

Birth control pills suppress eggs leaving the ovary and alter the hormone that causes the lining of the uterus to grow. Women who take birth control pills may experience sparse periods as a result of a decreased amount of uterine lining growth or increased bleeding due to changes in the hormone level. While scant bleeding is quite normal, heavy bleeding should not continue beyond two months. Report to your doctor any heavy bleeding that soaks more than one pad every two hours.

Heavy menstrual bleeding can occur from common, usually noncancerous tumors of the wall of the uterus (fibroid tumors, or leiomyomata). These tumors can compress the blood vessels in the wall of the uterus and distort them, prompting heavy vaginal bleeding. They often must be removed because they cause abnormal vaginal bleeding or severe pain, or because they become so large that they press on other organs, such as the bladder or rectum. There are also medications that may shrink these tumors.

Fortunately most abnormal vaginal bleeding, whether too much or too long, is not due to cancer. Usually the cause is noncancerous and treatable. However, seek medical evaluation by your doctor as soon as possible, because even certain noncancerous growths can turn into cancer. Also, continued blood loss can cause a dangerously low blood count (anemia), which may require blood transfusion or treatment with iron.

Tip 126:

If you have irregular menses or miss your periods, and/or have fluid leaking from engorged breasts, and you are not pregnant, you may have a tumor of the pituitary gland, which is located on the undersurface of your brain. This tumor may also limit your peripheral vision.

The following signs may be indicative of a tumor of the pituitary gland:

1. **A sudden abnormal change in your usual pattern of menstruation,** for example, missing periods for several months (when not pregnant).
2. **A feeling of "fullness" in your breasts** or a milky white discharge from your nipples (when not pregnant).

3. **Limitations in peripheral vision.** You cannot see objects coming from either side when you are looking straight ahead. Your vision is like the vision of a horse wearing blinders (see Tip 17).
4. **The onset of puberty before the age of nine.**

The pituitary gland produces hormones that regulate many other glands in the body. A pituitary tumor alters production of these hormones. This often results in changes in the activity of the glands that the pituitary gland regulates, such as the ovaries, which drive the menstrual cycle, and the breasts, which produce milk.

The above signs are an indication that a tumor may be growing in the pituitary gland. Early medical evaluation and treatment can cure this abnormal growth. A high level of prolactin, a hormone produced by the pituitary gland, suggests a tumor.

Shingles (a painful rash caused by a virus), sexual foreplay with the nipples, hypothyroidism (low thyroid gland function), and medications such as Thorazine and oral contraceptives can also cause nipple discharge.

•

Missed Periods

Tip 127:

Prolonged failure to menstruate in the absence of pregnancy usually means failure of one of the glands or part of the brain involved in providing a normal menstrual cycle. It is important to determine if there is a serious underlying cause.

When the egg bursts from the ovary (ovulation), it leaves behind a fluid collection (corpus luteum cyst) that produces hormones. These hormones make the lining of the uterus grow, preparing it to accept the fertilized egg. If fertilization does not occur, the lining of the uterus is shed (menstruation), and the cycle begins again. The menstrual flow consists of the shedding of the lining of the uterus (womb) mixed with blood.

If any of the above events fail to take place, the lining of the uterus will not grow, the lining will not be cast off, and there will be no period or menstruation. Glands other than the ovary are also involved in providing a normal menstrual cycle. Failure or abnormal function of these glands, which may be due to cancerous growths in the glands, can cause missed periods. Therefore prolonged failure to menstruate may be a sign that serious gland problems exist. Menstrual periods can be reinstituted with birth control pills, but it is still important to determine the underlying cause so that it can be treated.

Other hormone problems (such as excess estrogen) can also lead to lack of ovulation. In this case the lining of the uterus will grow, but there is no shedding or menstruation. Accumulation of the lining of the uterus may lead to cancer growth as early as six months from the time you start missing periods. Lack of ovulation is also a common cause of infertility. However, you can fail to menstruate, have a negative pregnancy test, and still have an ectopic pregnancy. (See Tip 181.)

Prolonged failure to menstruate without pregnancy requires timely medical evaluation, as do girls over the age of fifteen who have never had a menstrual period to determine the underlying cause and implement appropriate therapy.

•

Pain and PMS

> **Tip 128:**
>
> **Painful menstruation and PMS are not serious disorders, but some of the drugs used to treat them can have life-threatening, addictive effects.**

Premenstrual syndrome (PMS) is a cycle of symptoms that may include a combination of the following: headache, breast swelling, bloating, and emotional symptoms. It may begin many days before a menstrual period. Menstrual pain appears to be caused by specific hormones called prostaglandins, which alter the muscle walls of the womb and its blood vessels. Specific over-the-counter medications (nonsteroidal anti-inflammatory drugs) including Ibuprofen and Naproxen stop the production of these prostaglandin hormones. Starting the medicine at the appropriate dosage a few days before your period is often very effective treatment for the pain. Your doctor may decide to prescribe a diuretic (water pill) to alleviate the swelling and/or an antidepressant, or hormones to treat the symptoms of PMS. Exercise, diet modifications, and stress reduction techniques may also improve PMS symptoms.

On the other hand, be aware that tranquilizers or narcotics taken on a regular basis are potentially addictive and can have a serious negative impact on your mental and physical well-being. Narcotics are not an effective way to treat either PMS symptoms or menstrual cramps because they do not affect the production of the prostaglandin hormones that are responsible for these symptoms.

•

Bleeding After Menopause

Tip 129:

Vaginal bleeding after menopause is a warning sign of possible cancer.

Menopause occurs normally in women around the age of 50. It signals the end of menstrual periods because the ovaries run out of eggs and stop producing the hormones necessary for menstruation (estrogen). The menstrual pattern may become irregular before it stops altogether (perimenopause). It also may be accompanied by hot flashes. During a hot flash you suddenly feel hot and may even break out in a sweat lasting for two to three minutes. When twelve consecutive periods are missed, you are in menopause, and any bleeding afterward is abnormal. The stage of menopause can be confirmed by certain blood studies, but often it is not necessary to do these tests.

Recurrent vaginal bleeding after menopause is abnormal and may be an early warning sign of cancer, especially endometrial cancer (cancer in the lining of the womb). When this occurs, you should seek prompt medical evaluation. Early diagnosis and treatment can improve your chances of survival.

The risk factors for developing endometrial cancer are:

1. Obesity
2. Menstruating at an early age
3. Not having children
4. Menopause occurring at a late age
5. Diabetes mellitus

Groin

Tip 130:

A bulge of tissue often located in the groin area or around the belly button may be a hernia. Hernias are potentially dangerous and usually warrant repair.

Hernias are most common at the belly button or in the groin. A hernia occurs when a hole opens up in the muscles that make up the belly wall or other muscular walls. Belly contents push through the hole, especially when the pressure inside the belly cavity increases with activities such as lifting, straining, coughing, and the like. The hole often gets larger over time, increasing the possibility of belly contents pushing through. If a segment of intestine pushes through the hole, it can become kinked so much that it blocks the flow of bowel contents. This kink may also cut off the blood supply to the bowel, which can cause gangrene (death of part of the bowel). This condition is potentially fatal and warrants emergency surgical treatment.

When a bulge is noted, it is important to determine if the contents inside the bulge can be pushed back in. As long as they can, no immediate danger exists, but you should still consult your doctor about possibly repairing the hernia before it gets larger. Should the bulge be stuck, especially if it is tender and painful, urgent medical evaluation is needed.

Hips, Buttocks, Legs, and Ankles

Hips, Buttocks, and Legs

> **Tip 131:**
>
> Red and blue discoloration, swelling, pain and tenderness in the groin or leg may indicate the presence of blood clots, which may travel to the lungs.

Irritation of the walls of the veins is a setup for blood clots, because the blood can back up in these vessels. The groin or leg swells and turns bluish (from stagnant unoxygenated blood), and a reddish color may be present (from the inflamed veins). The back of the lower leg often hurts and is tender to touch. Phlebitis means "inflammation of veins."

There are many causes of phlebitis, including (1) the pooling of blood in the legs along with certain dilated and damaged veins near the surface of the skin (varicose veins); (2) an injury to the leg; (3) sitting for long periods of time (often during a trip in a car or airplane); (4) lying in bed for an extended period of time (bedridden at home or in the hospital); (5) cancer of the lung, colon, or blood, which may produce chemicals that attack the veins of the legs and cause phlebitis (this may be the first indication that a cancer exists), and (6) a generalized inflammation of blood vessels that develops with diseases of the connective tissue, such as lupus.

Phlebitis is potentially deadly because a piece of the clot in a vein of the leg might break off and travel through the blood vessels, resulting in a large life-threatening clot in the lungs. A clot in the lungs produces shortness of breath and an inability to oxygenate the blood. (See Tips 52 and 74.) Therefore it is urgent that you see a doctor for evaluation and treatment, including a blood thinner if appropriate.

Tip 132:

Pain in your legs, hips, and/or buttocks when you walk may result not from arthritis but from clogged arteries in your legs. When the blockage of the arteries is total, gangrene of the leg and infection can occur. The infection may spread to the rest of your body.

Pain in the legs during activities such as walking, which is relieved during rest, is usually due to insufficient blood flow to the legs. During activity the leg muscles require more blood. When they do not receive it, you feel pain in these muscles. The distance you can walk before the pain occurs is determined by the degree of blockage in the artery to your leg. A severe blockage may bring on the pain after walking only a few feet. Less severe blockage may allow walking for a quarter of a mile. Rarely the pain occurs at the first attempt to walk but then disappears as you walk for a while. This is unusual, however.

If the blockage is in the arteries of the thighs, the pain is in the calves. Higher blockage will cause pain in the hips, buttocks, and thighs.

If a blood clot forms in the markedly narrowed area of the artery, a complete blockage of the artery will follow, with severe leg pain. When this occurs, there is danger of losing the leg. If the blood flow has been interrupted for too long, causing gangrene with the risk of a life-threatening infection spreading throughout the body, amputation is necessary.

If you experience pain in your leg when you walk, you should seek medical evaluation as soon as possible. It is best to correct the problem before total blockage occurs. Circulation may be restored by cleaning out the blockage. The artery can be reopened with a small tube with an inflatable balloon, to open the narrowed area. Surgical repair is also possible. One end of a small piece of vessel is sewn to the blocked vessel above the site of the obstruction, while the other end is sewn below the site of the blockage. This allows blood to bypass or detour around the site of the obstruction. A third approach is to inject a substance in the blood vessel that can dissolve the blood clot.

Tip 133:

Bone pain that wakes you in the middle of the night may be cancer originating in the bone.

Deep, aching pains in the bones, the kind that wake you up in the middle of the night, could be a sign of cancer. You need to distinguish it from pains in the joints, which are usually due to arthritis.

Cancer originating in the bone can involve the bone itself or the core of the bone where blood cells are made.

If you suffer from severe bone pain, an early visit to your doctor for evaluation and treatment may result in a cure.

•

Ankles

Tip 134:

General swelling of the ankles can be the sign of a serious disease.

Standing too long causes swelling of the ankles, especially if you are overweight or pregnant. If this is the cause, the swelling is not significant and clears after a night of rest. On the other hand, lower leg swelling may also be an important sign of a serious disease, including inflamed or blocked varicose veins. It may occur if you have heart, liver, and kidney disease, a low-functioning thyroid gland, cancer elsewhere in the body, or side effects of medication.

You may have lower leg swelling and not even know it. To test for it, stand up for a while, press your thumb firmly over your shinbone for five to ten seconds, then release it. If the imprint of the thumb remains, significant swelling is present. The deeper the pit, the worse the swelling. If the swelling does not disappear after one night of rest or leg elevation, it is important to seek medical evaluation.

Skin

Bites

Tip 135:

The bite of an animal with rabies can be fatal. Therefore, if you are bitten by a dog, cat, raccoon, fox, skunk, bat, or certain other animals, immediate medical attention is necessary. Also, you can get rabies from exposure to the saliva of a rabid animal. Bats flying in the room of a sleeping person or near an awake, unattended child have been reported to infect the individual with no known bite.

Animals with rabies, including dogs, cats, horses, bats, foxes, and raccoons, can give you rabies if they bite you. The rabies virus can also be transferred if the animal's saliva comes in contact with your mucous membranes, for example, in your mouth. If you take immunization shots, you can avoid developing the disease.

Fortunately the time of exposure to the appearance of symptoms is approximately one month. The animal should be observed for ten days, and if it begins to act strangely, it should be tested for rabies. If the animal is found to have rabies, you will need the rabies immunization.

Rabies immunization involves receiving a series of shots. This is necessary since untreated rabies is almost 100 percent fatal.

If the animal is not captured and observed, your physician will have to use his or her best judgment to determine whether to start the immunization shots.

Tip 136:

If you have had a severe allergic reaction, the next time it could be worse—even life-threatening. Swelling of the lips and throat, and/or difficulty breathing after a beesting or exposure to another allergen are red light warning signals. See Tip 160 if you are currently experiencing these symptoms.

Serious allergic reactions can get worse with every episode. Each time exposure occurs, vital areas of the body can become more sensitized, resulting in more severe reactions with subsequent exposure. Such sensitization can lead to massive swelling, with closure of the windpipe, shock, and death.

If there is any possibility that you might be at risk of

a severe allergic reaction to any biting or stinging insect, food, cosmetic, plant, dye, and so on, carry an emergency treatment kit with you at all times (see Tip 160). An immediate shot of adrenaline after a life-threatening reaction, with sudden shortness of breath, wheezes, and weakness, could save your life. Some treatments reduce the severity of these allergic reactions. Consult with your doctor or an allergist.

Tip 137:

Human bites are serious. The bitten area can become infected, requiring treatment by a physician.

There are more germs in the human mouth than in the mouth of a dog. Therefore if the teeth of a human go through your skin, watch out, even if it is a cut in your hand that results from a punch to a person's mouth. For the first forty-eight hours after the bite, the wound may not look bad. Later, redness and swelling may appear, followed by pus. Immediate antiseptic cleansing and removal of damaged tissue from the wound at the time of injury by a health professional can prevent the spread of infection. Also, get a tetanus shot if you haven't received one in the past ten years.

Tip 138:

If you are bitten by a poisonous snake, antivenom shots may save your life.

After a snakebite, examination of the snake (dead or alive) can determine if it is poisonous. This can help the doctor decide what treatment is necessary. If possible, bring any remnants of the snake to the doctor's office. But do not attempt to capture or kill the snake if it puts you in danger of another bite.

If the snake's poison gets into your bloodstream, death may be sudden unless you can get immediate treatment with antivenom shots. It is always urgent to seek immediate medical evaluation if you have been bitten by a poisonous snake.

The following steps should be taken at the time you are bitten, if it won't cause excessive delay in getting you to medical care:

1. Stay calm.
2. Try not to move the area that has been bitten.
3. Wipe the wound with a clean cloth to remove poison left on the skin.
4. Do not apply a tourniquet, cut open the bite, suction or tamper with the wound in any way.
5. Seek emergency medical care.

Tip 139:

The bite of a tick can cause you to stagger, become uncoordinated, or even cause paralysis, which usually clears when the tick is removed.

A tick bite on the back of the neck near the base of the skull can cause "tick paralysis." The tick attaches, burrows its head through the skin, feeds on your blood, and regurgitates a toxin into your skin. If the tick is removed, the paralysis often clears.

If you stagger and become uncoordinated for no apparent reason, examine the back of your neck and other parts of your body for a tick. Seek immediate medical evaluation and treatment. It is important to have the entire tick removed. The tick can be removed by putting alcohol on the tick to relax it. The skin is stretched and the tick is pulled off with tweezers.

●

Discolorations

Tip 140:

Changes in your pattern of bruising, little black or red dots on your skin, nosebleeds, gum bleeds, rectal bleeding, or bleeding too long after a cut may indicate blood-clotting problems from an ailment or the side effect of a medication (such as aspirin or certain over-the-counter or prescription pain pills).

If your normal pattern of bruising changes, you may have a serious problem with the clotting of your blood. Other signs of clotting problems include little black or red dots (pin-sized bleeding spots on the skin), nosebleeds, gum bleeding, and rectal bleeding.

Blood clotting requires a cascade of many different chemical reactions. If any of the factors involved are missing, your blood may not clot normally. Hemophiliacs are born without a specific clotting factor and need a replacement. Certain clotting substances are made in the liver; therefore if you have a liver ailment, you may bleed more easily.

Particles in your blood (called platelets) prevent blood from leaking out of the tiny blood vessels (capillaries). Platelets also release chemicals that aid in the clotting process. If you begin to bruise or bleed easily, it could be a result of a low platelet level. Low platelets can be a side effect of a medication you are taking (such as aspirin, certain over-the-counter or prescription pain pills in the NSAID category) or the result of a disease that destroys platelets, such as an enlarged spleen or hemolytic uremic syndrome more commonly seen in children. (See Tip 203.)

This condition needs immediate medical attention, since it places you at a higher risk of bleeding in your brain (a stroke) or bleeding internally at some other site in your body.

Tip 141:

A darkening and thickening of the skin around the back of the neck, armpits, and groin of an adult (usually over 40) can be a sign of cancer or diabetes.

If you notice that your skin is darker than your normal skin color in places such as the back of the neck, the armpits, or the groin area, you may have a condition known as acanthosis nigricans. The skin condition itself is harmless, and it may not be associated with any disease. But it can also be a sign of a disease such as can-

cer of the stomach or colon. It is also found in obese
people with high levels of the hormone insulin who are
at risk of developing diabetes. Weight reduction may
improve this condition. It is more common in dark-
skinned individuals.

If you have this condition, you should see your physician for an evaluation to determine if you have any of
the serious associated diseases.

Tip 142:

**Dark spots (brown in African Americans and
Asians, pink to dusty red in Caucasians) on the
palms of the hands may be a sign of syphilis or
Rocky Mountain spotted fever. If treated early, fatal
heart and brain complications can be avoided.**

The appearance of dark spots all over the palms of
your hands—spots that do not itch or hurt—is a red
light warning signal. Unlike blisterlike raised bumps on
the skin that peel and itch, these spots do not break the
surface of the skin.

Two unrelated infectious diseases can cause this
sign: syphilis and Rocky Mountain spotted fever.
Rocky Mountain spotted fever, caused by a bacteria-
like germ transmitted by a tick bite, is accompanied
by a high fever and severe headache. (See Tip 153
for additional discussion concerning Rocky Mountain
spotted fever.) On the other hand, the syphilis
germ could be living in your body without any symptoms. Urgent treatment of either ailment can be lifesaving.

Tip 143:

Turning blue often indicates an insufficient oxygen supply. It is commonly seen in children with inherited heart abnormalities and people with breathing problems. It can also occur as a side effect of certain medicines and from other causes. If your skin turns blue, you need immediate medical evaluation and possible treatment.

Most people think that when the skin turns blue, it is from an inability to breathe. It is true that cutting off your oxygen supply will make you turn blue in a hurry. But there are other reasons, too, why your skin might turn blue.

Normally oxygen attaches to a protein called hemoglobin in your red blood cells. This occurs as blood travels through the blood vessels in your lungs. The oxygen is then transported throughout the body for use by all the body's organs. This gives a normal pink color to the skin of Caucasians and to the mucous membranes (the lining of the mouth, nose, eyes, and so on) of all people. If the oxygen supply to the blood is cut off for any reason, the hemoglobin circulates without oxygen. This gives the skin a blue appearance (cyanosis).

Many ailments can decrease the oxygenation of the blood, including inherited heart abnormalities in children as well as lung disease. In addition, certain medications and maladies can sometimes alter the hemoglobin in some of the red blood cells so that they are unable to carry oxygen, which also turns your skin a bluish color.

If your skin and/or lips turns blue, you need to be

evaluated by a doctor immediately to determine the underlying cause. Your body organs may not be receiving sufficient oxygen, which can have a long-term negative effect on your health. In many cases therapeutic intervention can reverse the disorder.

Tip 144:

A low count of red blood cells (anemia) can cause paleness, fatigue, and a rapid pulse with or without shortness of breath. In certain cases you may feel dizzy or pass out. Diagnosing and treating causes of a low blood count can be lifesaving.

There are many reasons why you could have a low blood count. They include (1) poor nutrition; (2) a disease that destroys the bone marrow, where red blood cells are made; (3) a drug that causes red blood cells to break apart; (4) cancer in the colon with a slow bleed; and (5) heavy menstrual flow. It is important to seek medical attention to diagnose the cause of a low blood count. In many cases early treatment can cure the underlying ailment.

If untreated, a very low blood count can result in serious damage to your organs. Red blood cells carry and supply oxygen to your brain and heart. When your blood count is dangerously low, an immediate blood transfusion can be lifesaving. The doctor can easily tell how low your blood count is by drawing a sample of your blood and performing a simple test. If you have symptoms of fatigue, shortness of breath, and/or pale skin, you should see a doctor right away to determine your blood count and for a thorough evaluation. If you also have a rapid pulse, the bleeding may be sudden, requiring immediate transport to an emergency room.

Tip 145:

If you notice a serious skin sensitivity to the sun, check the side effects of the medicines you are taking. Also certain diseases such as lupus can cause skin sensitivity to the sun.

Hundreds of medicines can make your skin sensitive to the sun. There are two main types of reactions:

1. **Phototoxic reaction.** This type of reaction occurs immediately because the medication causes the skin to be much more sensitive to the ultraviolet light of the sun. This can cause such sun sensitivity that a normally harmless amount of sunlight may burn your skin.
2. **Photoallergic reaction.** This type of reaction is due to an allergic sensitization of the skin by a drug. (It appears after being on the medicine awhile, even as long as a few weeks.) Skin exposed to the sun may develop eczema, hives, small fine bumps, hard plaques, or blisters. These reactions may continue to recur for some time after the drug has been discontinued.

Since so many different medicines can cause these reactions, consult your doctor or pharmacist to determine if a drug you are taking has these side effects. You can ask the pharmacist for a copy of the package insert to see if skin sensitivity to the sun is a side effect. These reactions can be very serious and even fatal, even in sun-tanning salons.

It is important to be aware of the potential side effects of all the medicines you take. If you develop a reaction, you should discuss it with your doctor as soon as possible to determine the safest way to deal with it (for example, by changing medicines). Don't make these decisions alone.

•

Freckles, Moles, Bumps, Warts, Lumps, Plaques, and Patches

Tip 146:

Irregular-shaped, dark, multicolored, enlarging, bleeding, itching, or painful moles need frequent checking for early detection of malignant melanoma. Early treatment can be lifesaving.

Moles that can turn into cancer (malignant melanoma) may be raised, like regular moles, or flush with the skin surface, like large, dark freckles. They often begin as an abnormal growth of pigment cells and darken with exposure to the sun. Pigmented lesions on the pads of the hands and soles of the feet are even more likely to turn into malignant melanomas. A rare type of melanoma has no pigment.

If you have a mole or moles with any of the following features (which suggest they are cancerous), see your doctor or a dermatologist right away:

1. Asymmetrical shape—not a smooth, round circle, like a regular mole
2. Multicolored appearance, with shades of brown, black, gray, red, and white
3. Large size (greater than the eraser end of a pencil)
4. Growth in size over a period of time, unlike regular moles, which do not grow
5. Itching, pain, or bleeding

The incidence of malignant melanomas is increasing in the population at large. They are most common in adults over 30 years of age and are the most common cancer in the 25-to-35 age group.

The following increase your risk of developing this cancer:

1. You have been diagnosed by a physician as having certain types of moles that are precancerous.
2. Members of your family have had a malignant melanoma.
3. You are light-skinned and easily sunburned.
4. You have been exposed to a great deal of sunlight, especially in childhood and adolescence, and have had multiple sunburns in the past.
5. You have many moles of any kind.

Monitor your moles on a regular basis, including those in the genital area where changes are often missed (the use of a mirror may be helpful). Avoid tanning beds. If you are at greater risk, your dermatologist or doctor should assist you in monitoring your moles. If you detect a suspicious mole see your doctor or dermatologist as soon as possible so it can be removed early and examined under a microscope.

Use sun protection routinely after six months of age. UVB and UVA sun protection factor (SPF) should be 30 or greater. The container should indicate that two types of light are blocked (UVB and UVA).

Tip 147:

A pearly bump on the face or other area of the skin exposed to the sun is a potential sign of skin cancer. Early treatment is important.

If you are a senior citizen, spend lots of time in the sun, and have developed a round, pearly bump on your face, you may have a skin cancer known as basal cell carcinoma. The face, like other areas of the skin exposed to sunlight, is a common site for this tumor. Basal cell cancers are usually slow growing and do not spread, but there are exceptions.

The diagnosis is made when your doctor cuts off a slice of the bump and looks at it under a microscope. Surgical removal can usually cure a basal cell carcinoma. If you suspect you may have skin cancer, do not wait. See your physician early.

Tip 148:

Freckles on the lips, in the mouth, or on the inside of the lips are associated with growths in the colon, which can become cancerous (Peutz-Jeghers syndrome).

In the unusual, inherited condition called Peutz-Jeghers syndrome, freckles occur on the lips and inside the mouth, in addition to dangerous polyps (growths) in the colon.

If you have this pattern of freckles, a colonoscopic exam by a doctor may be appropriate to find any polyps and remove them, if possible, to avoid bleeding and prevent a cancerous growth. Sometimes these growths can be malignant, in which case early surgical removal can be curative.

Let your doctor know if you develop this red light warning signal. (See Tip 215 for more information on this disorder in children.)

Tip 149:

A yellow, cheesy-looking plaque in the skin above or under an eye, or in another area of your skin, can mean you have a high level of cholesterol in your blood, which can be life-threatening.

A yellow, cheesy-looking plaque, usually about a quarter of an inch wide, may appear above or under your eye or at the side of your nose. Occasionally it appears under the elbow or in another location on the skin. It is oblong in shape, not round like a cyst. It usually does not cause discomfort. You cannot squeeze out the contents because the plaque is within your skin. This plaque is probably a cholesterol deposit.

A cholesterol deposit may be a warning sign that you have a dangerously high blood cholesterol level. This cholesterol can invade the wall of an artery. Eventually it can result in total blockage of vital blood vessels that provide nourishment to the heart or brain, causing a heart attack or stroke.

These yellow, cheesy-looking plaques are a warning message that you should heed. See your doctor and have your cholesterol and other blood fat levels checked. These plaques can be removed for cosmetic reasons, but they may recur. But most importantly, high cholesterol and other fat levels in the blood should be lowered with diet and/or medicines. (See Tip 165 for more information on an elevated cholesterol level, especially in senior citizens.)

•

Infections

Tip 150:

Occasionally an infection on the skin can spread very rapidly often causing red streaks. It can be fatal.

A wound that has become infected with germs is red and slightly swollen. Infected cuts or abrasions are common and, if kept clean, get better in twenty-four hours. But if the redness of an infection spreads and there is more swelling and pain, watch out. Certain nasty germs, such as streptococci and staphylococci, can spread rapidly. Red streaks running up the arm or leg from the site of the infection indicates a rapid and dangerous spread of germs.

If your infected wound is getting worse, consult your physician immediately. Your doctor can swab (culture) the infected site, examine it to detect the kind of germ, and determine which specific antibiotic will effectively kill it.

•

Itchy Skin

Tip 151:

Itching all over without a sign of a rash can indicate cancer, liver disease, kidney disease, a psychological problem, or other illness, as well as a potentially serious reaction to a medication.

Most of the time itching skin, such as dry skin, has an obvious explanation. But itching all over (without rash) can be an early sign of cancer, including lymphoma and leukemia, often associated with a low-grade fever. Diffuse itching from an accumulation of substances normally broken down in the liver may be the first sign of liver disease. Infection, kidney disease, psychological disorders, and blood and glandular illnesses, as well as side effects of drugs, can cause itching.

Therefore itching all over your skin may appropriately indicate a need for a thorough medical checkup. If it is a sudden onset, particularly after taking medicine, notify your doctor before continuing your medications, since it could be an early sign of a life-threatening aller-

gic reaction. This may occur when you take the second
dose.

•

Rashes

Tip 152:

A bull's-eye red rash, with or without joint pain,
is a sign of Lyme disease from a tick bite.

The initial event in Lyme disease is a skin rash: a red-
dened area, circular in shape, with more intense redness
at the center. It gives the overall appearance of a bull's-
eye. The rash itself will clear up without treatment, but
the disease will spread to other areas of the body.
Initially you may have flu-type symptoms and/or a fever.
As the disease progresses, you may develop joint pain,
weakness, and tiredness. Eventually the brain and heart
will be damaged.

If you have this type of rash, contact your doctor
immediately. Treatment of Lyme disease with antibiotics
during the rash phase is very effective and will usually
cure it. When the infection spreads to other parts of the
body, treatment is more complicated. Chronic Lyme disease can be a very disabling illness.

Although Lyme disease is not very common, it
does pose a threat, especially along the Atlantic coast
and Midwest. The tick that transmits the disease
is smaller than most, so the tick bite often goes unnoticed.

Tip 153:

Tick bites transmit Rocky Mountain spotted fever, which is identified by a high fever and a rash on the palms of the hands and the soles of the feet. You will reduce your risk if you use insect repellent and remove the ticks from your body after each day spent in the woods.

Some ticks carry the Rocky Mountain spotted fever germ. These organisms gain entrance to the body through the bite of a tick, then spread throughout the body. After about ten days you develop a high fever, weakness, chills, a headache, and a generalized flat rash. Little pinpoint blood spots appear. The rash, which involves the palms of the hands and soles of the feet, usually does not occur in other acute illnesses associated with a fever. Since this disease can be fatal, immediate medical attention is necessary, even if the tick is not found.

Ticks need time to spread disease, so check your body for ticks immediately after you return from the woods. Dousing a cotton ball with rubbing alcohol and holding it over the tick will relax the creature so that you can pluck it off your skin safely with a pair of tweezers. Make certain you remove the entire tick.

Tip 154:

Everyone with hives (an intensely itching, giant mosquito bite–appearing rash) ought to have at least one medical evaluation, because hives can occur with blood cancers.

Hives are common and appear as a widespread, raised, red, itchy, swollen rash that may look like giant mosquito bites. Most commonly they are a result of a generalized allergic reaction to foods, pollen, or medicines. Exposure to heat and cold, sunlight, stress, and infections can also influence the development of hives.

The most frustrating feature of hives is its recurring nature. Once it gets rolling, it may improve and then pop out again a few days later, without known reexposure to any precipitating factor.

Certain blood-borne and other cancers can cause hives, such as leukemia and cancer of the lymph system. Although this rarely occurs, it is advisable to be checked out by your physician, who may do more extensive testing if he or she is suspicious that a serious condition is causing the hives. (Also see Tips 160 and 145.)

•

Sores

Tip 155:

If you have had a draining sore for months, and it will not heal, particularly if it is on your neck, your forearm, or your foot, you may have a serious body-invading fungus infection. There are many other treatable causes of nonhealing sores that also require immediate medical evaluation and treatment.

Fungus infections are always life-threatening in persons with impaired immune systems. Most of them are limited to the skin and nails. Some can invade the body and spread to the internal organs. It is important to see your doctor as soon as possible for tests on the material draining from the wound so early treatment can be instituted.

The most common presentation of a fungus infection is a rash. In those with an impaired immune system, a deep draining sore that does not heal is more common. The most common sites are the neck, usually around the angle of the jaw, the forearm, and the foot.

Yeast infections are also fungal. They are usually confined to the vagina, around the corners of the mouth, or in the mouth. A life-threatening blood-borne yeast infection is more common among patients with poor defense mechanisms, including people with AIDS, people who are receiving chemotherapy for cancer, and people taking steroids and other drugs after receiving an organ transplant. Yeast infections are usually responsive to an antifungal antibiotic.

Tip 156:

An ulcer on the skin that does not heal after a maximum of one month could be skin cancer and needs to be evaluated.

Occasionally people attribute a sore or ulcer that does not heal to an injury, when actually it was not caused by trauma. Any ulcer that does not heal within a maximum of one month should be evaluated by a doctor to rule out cancer or an underlying disease.

•

Back

Back Pain

Tip 157:

Back pain that originates just above the belt line, three to four inches on either side of the center of the back, indicates kidney disease that may need immediate medical attention. Often the pain is associated with fever and urination problems and is made worse when you gently tap the area.

The kidneys are located just above the belt line, three to four inches on either side of the middle of the back. The back pain is often but not necessarily accompanied by fever and/or pain and difficulty urinating. It is more likely to occur on the sides of the back and in the abdomen than exclusively in the center of the lower back (see Figure 13). The back pain is often made worse by tapping on the area.

It is important that you seek medical evaluation and treatment for this type of back pain as soon as possible. Many types of kidney disease can get worse over time. With proper treatment the ailment can often be cured or at least prevented from getting worse. (See Tip 122 for more information on evaluation and treatment of urinary tract infections.)

Tip 158:

The sudden onset of severe back pain could be a compression fracture, which occurs when there is general weakness in the bones caused by loss of the thickness or mass of bones. It is more common in senior citizens and requires more bed rest than normal. Sedentary older people are at a high risk of developing blood clots and infection. An objective is to avoid fractures in the first place.

Sudden agonizing back pain can be the result of a softening of the bones (osteoporosis) and a vertebral fracture. Weak bones are more susceptible to fractures and collapse.

Osteoporosis develops gradually and usually without symptoms. It often begins in older women at the onset of menopause, since the ovaries produce less estrogen, resulting in the bones losing more calcium. It also can begin earlier in life, depending on such factors

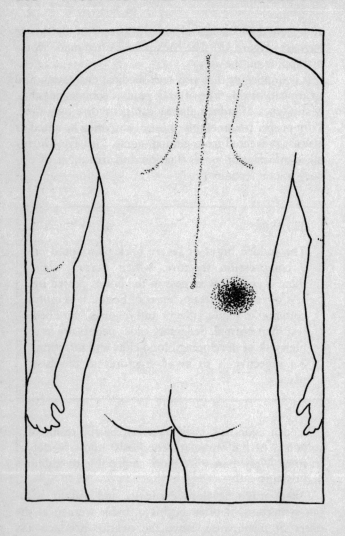

Figure 13. Kidney Pain.

as body weight, degree of physical activity, and genetic factors.

Bones that bear weight, such as the vertebrae of the spine, are the first to experience a change from the softening. The weight of the body causes the framework of the vertebrae to gradually break down and compress. This process causes older people to lose height. If a vertebra collapses (compression fracture), it can produce agonizing pain.

Confinement to bed, often resulting from fractures of the spine, hips, and legs, is the enemy of the senior citizen, as it may lead to early death from blood clots or infections in the lungs. Lying still creates an environment where blood is more stagnant and more likely to clot. Therefore early activity with a brace is often recommended.

New treatment options are available to increase the thickness (mass) of the bones and thus strengthen them. This preventive therapy may be appropriate for those with osteoporosis. But the side effects and costs of the treatment must be considered before starting it. If you have osteoporosis, you should discuss the pros and cons of this therapy with your physician.

Tip 159:

Severe back and leg pain, especially when accompanied by fever, may mean you have a serious infection rather than a backbone problem such as a disk herniation or spur.

You have a cut on your leg with some nasty-looking redness around it, which appears to be a minor infection. Or you have pain during urination, or a chest cold that seems to be getting worse. Then you develop an overwhelming, agonizing severe pain in your lower back and legs. Your temperature may rise. The pain is so severe that you don't mention the associated symptoms when you call your doctor—they seem so minor. The doctor can easily assume your back pain is caused by a run-of-the-mill muscle strain or lumbar disk disease and make the wrong diagnosis.

This error can have dire consequences. Though it happens rarely, minor infections can rapidly spread through the bloodstream to many locations in the body. Fever and severe back pain, frequently accompanied by leg pain, may be the signal. Sometimes if a massive infection overwhelms the body's defense mechanism, there is no fever. Immediate treatment by a doctor is crucial, which includes intravenous antibiotics to save the patient's life. Senior citizens and/or debilitated people are more vulnerable to these massive infections. An important message here is to always carefully report all symptoms of an ailment to the doctor, even if you feel they are minor.

PART TWO

•

General Symptoms and Signs (More Common in Adults): Not Body Part–Specific Conditions

Allergic Reactions

Tip 160:

A serious, life-threatening allergic reaction, especially starting with a swollen tongue, or lips, or throat and breathing problems, may progress rapidly, within minutes. It can be reversed if medical treatment is started immediately.

Allergic reactions are common. They can follow exposure to about anything, but they usually occur from foods, certain plants, beestings, or medicines. Allergic reactions are not dose related—you can have a serious reaction to even a tiny exposure. And you can develop allergic reactions to things you were not allergic to in the past.

Most allergic reactions result only in an itchy rash and swelling. Occasionally the swelling will become severe when it occurs in locations of loose skin around the eyes or groin. This massive swelling looks bad but is usually not dangerous. It responds well to medical treatment.

Rarely allergic reactions occur very rapidly and become life-threatening. The main cause of death in severe allergic reactions is the inability to breathe because of a blockage of the airways and collapse of blood pressure from a sudden dilation (expansion) of blood vessels throughout the body.

To prevent the serious consequences, know the early symptoms. Immediate treatment can save your life. You are in danger of a full-blown allergic reaction and need to get to an emergency room immediately, or need to receive an epinephrine shot on the spot, if you have the following symptoms within thirty minutes of exposure:

1. Swelling of the tongue and mouth
2. Hoarseness, a "lump in the throat" feeling, difficulty swallowing
3. Breathing problems, a cough, chest tightness, wheezing, and croup
4. Dizziness, with a cold sweat and/or profuse sweating
5. Abdominal cramps and/or vomiting
6. A loss of consciousness

Be prepared! If you have had a severe allergic reaction in the past, it may be worse the next time, so ask your doctor for a home epinephrine kit. The kit contains a single shot of the drug epinephrine, which you can inject into your muscle. The medicine opens your airways and tightens your blood vessels.

To prevent allergic reactions, first become familiar with your allergies. Make a record of all allergic reactions you have experienced and what caused them. The following are some of the most common substances (allergens) to which people are allergic:

1. Foods: shellfish, soybeans, nuts, milk, eggs, MSG, sulfites
2. Insect bites: bees, wasps, ants
3. Drugs: penicillin (most common), aspirin, sulfa-based drugs, ibuprofen or other nonaspirin pain medicine
4. Radiographic contrast material: the fluid injected into you during a study such as a CT scan (a special computerized X-ray), an IVP (a special X-ray of your kidney), angiography (special X-ray study of your arteries), etc.

Once you have identified your exact allergens, which may require testing by an allergist, try to avoid exposure to them. Inform your physician of all your allergies, especially to drugs or to contrast material injected into you during X-ray procedures. Consider purchasing an engraved bracelet listing your allergens. Ask your pharmacist where to obtain one of these bracelets. It can be useful in emergency situations.

An allergist is a medical specialist who can help you identify your specific allergies and, if you have the potential of a serious reaction, help you prevent them.

There is a rare but potentially fatal ailment similar to an allergic reaction. It is called angioedema. The red light warning signals are isolated painless swelling of either the tongue, mouth, lip, usually one hand or one foot, etc., without itching. People with this condition can spontaneously develop swelling in the windpipe, cutting off their air supply. These swellings are rare and often occur for no known reason. They have also been associated with the blood pressure and heart medications known as ACE inhibitors (check with your pharmacist or doctor to determine if any of the medications you are taking fall into this category). Urgent evaluation and treatment of this type of swelling is necessary. (See Tip 220 for more information on allergies.)

Tip 161:

Allergic reactions to medication commonly occur in the form of a rash or upset stomach. Other symptoms include a low-grade fever, aching joints and muscles, and a sore mouth and tongue. Rarely, life-threatening reactions occur.

The most common type of medication reaction is an allergic reaction, such as a skin rash. The rash usually itches, and its appearance varies from patches of small red bumps to hives. The rash may occur anywhere on the body. Usually the reaction does not result in serious complications if the medication is stopped (after consultation with your doctor, to make sure it is safe to do so). Your doctor can prescribe treatments to alleviate symptoms. The rare severe reactions usually occur immediately after starting or restarting a medication. In life-threatening situations associated with weakness, shortness of breath, wheezing, vomiting, and/or dizziness, emergency epinephrine shots are necessary.

Another common reaction to medication is a sore tongue or mouth. Anytime this occurs, it should be considered a medication reaction until proven otherwise. Reactions occur from prescription medicines as well as over-the-counter medications, including headache pills, aspirin, laxatives, or sinus pills.

You may also experience stomach irritation in reaction to a medication. This is quite common with over-the-counter pain medicines. Make sure you notify your doctor and stop the medicine because stomach ulceration can occur—it can lead to a life-threatening hemorrhage. (For more information see Tip 93.)

Sometimes initial symptoms may be quite vague. You gradually become more fatigued, you develop a low-grade fever, and you ache all over. It sounds like the flu. But after a week your condition worsens. It is time to go back to the doctor because you may have developed a severe toxic effect from the medication.

Many medications can ultimately cause a severe inflammatory reaction in the kidneys, which could lead to kidney failure, or a reaction in the liver, which could lead to a chemical hepatitis and liver failure. It is prudent to be on the lookout for this phenomenon when starting a new medication. Always consult your physician immediately if you think a medication is causing any of these effects.

In addition, review the package insert available from your pharmacist, for side effects relating to all the medications you are taking.

Tip 162:

On rare occasions certain medications can cause fatal reactions, starting with a targetlike (usually dark spots with a pale center) rash usually with a low-grade fever. It is treatable and curable if caught early.

Although rarely certain medications can cause rashes that may lead to death. It sounds unbelievable that a rash alone could be a warning sign. You will know if you are having a reaction by the presence of a targetlike rash on your skin, sometimes followed by a low-grade fever, redness and soreness in the mouth, throat, and/or eyes. Left untreated, this condition can develop into Stevens-Johnson syndrome, a severe allergic reaction that may damage a large amount of the skin, causing it to slough off. When it develops, fatalities are frequent. Therefore early diagnosis and treatment are essential. If you develop a targetlike rash after starting certain medications, get to a doctor immediately.

Tip 163:

Although very rare, increasing weakness in the arms and legs, and/or changes in your ability to feel pressure or heat, can lead to paralysis and death following certain infections, and possibly a vaccination, such as influenza.

Guillain-Barré syndrome is an ailment consisting of weakness in the arms and legs that may progress throughout the body. It is also associated with a loss of ability to feel pressure or heat. An allergic reaction and/or inflammation initially occurs in the nerves. It gradually interrupts the transmission of nerve impulses to the areas of the body controlled by these nerves. This results in the gradual onset of paralysis in the arms and legs (usually starting from the toes or fingers and moving up the body), with increasing difficulty in breathing. Death may occur if medical treatment is not instituted. Most people recover with proper treatment, but rehabilitation is lengthy. One form of treatment is plasma-pheresis, a process that cleans the blood of bound antibodies formed during the allergic reaction. If this procedure is done before the muscles for breathing are affected, it may prevent you from being put on a ventilator.

If weakness of your arms and legs occurs, see your doctor immediately, or get to an emergency room.

Blood and Blood Pressure

Tip 164:

Even a mild elevation in blood pressure can put you at risk of having a heart attack, stroke, kidney disease, or heart failure.

It is a common misconception that mild high blood pressure (hypertension) is not serious. Optimal blood pressure is 120 over 80 or less. If the upper number (the systolic blood pressure) is above 120 or the lower number (the diastolic blood pressure) is above 80, you are at a higher risk of stroke, heart disease, and kidney failure than those with a lower blood pressure. Mild to moderate elevations do not usually cause noticeable symptoms, but they are still dangerous to your health. Hypertension is known as a "silent killer." Slight elevations such as 160 over 90 often are ignored for months or years, which is a mistake. Even these slight elevations can cause damage to the heart, brain, or kidneys, eventually resulting in a stroke, kidney failure, heart attack, or heart failure at an early age.

Any elevation should be monitored with repeated blood pressure recordings. You should be evaluated by a doctor to determine the most effective therapeutic approach for controlling your blood pressure.

Tip 165:

Treatment of high cholesterol and other abnormal blood lipids (fats) is important, even if you are a senior citizen.

Elevated cholesterol and other blood fats can create fatty deposits (plaques) that block arteries, which may result in a heart attack or stroke. These plaques can also create blockages in the blood vessels of the legs. Many people think that the time to diet and/or take medication to prevent this is when you are young. Often senior citizens believe that the damage is done and there's nothing they can do about it. This is absolutely wrong.

Recently microscopic photographs taken inside arteries show that cholesterol deposits can shrink or even disappear with treatment. Originally it was thought that the gradual buildup of fats in its walls would totally block an artery, at which point no more blood would pass through the vessel. If it is a blood vessel supplying the heart with nourishment, a heart attack can result. On the other hand, if it is an artery supplying the brain with nourishment, a stroke with paralysis can result.

But recent research indicates that the fat does not

totally block the blood vessel. It blocks it only partially. Total blockage is actually caused by a chemical reaction at the site of the fatty deposit, resulting in the formation of a blood clot. Therefore if you shrink the fatty deposits, the likelihood of blood clotting diminishes, reducing the incidence of heart attack and stroke. This is confirmed by the scientific finding that both young and old people live longer after lowering their cholesterol and other blood fat levels.

The medications now used in the treatment of these problems are very effective. Liver toxicity from some of these medicines is very rare and most people have no problem with this side effect. Your doctor can monitor your liver function with certain blood tests.

Tip 166:

The best method to control blood spurting from a blood vessel due to a severe laceration is direct pressure. This approach is better than using a tourniquet.

Very few things are more frightening than seeing blood spurting from a severed artery after a serious injury. You know you need to reduce the bleeding, but what is the best method? It is best accomplished by direct pressure, using whatever is available. Ideally, gauze dressing is applied and firmly pressed against the wound. If gauze is not available, any type of cloth material will suffice. Continued compression will cause the artery to constrict and clotting will follow. Even bleeding from a large artery can be controlled in this fashion until emergency care arrives. If you are assisting an injured person, avoid contaminating your eyes, mouth, or an open wound with the blood. Wear gloves when available and wash yourself well for fifteen minutes as soon as possible.

Tip 167:

Low potassium levels in the blood can make you feel very weak and cause muscle cramps. It can also cause a fatal heart rhythm problem. High potassium can also cause muscle weakness and serious heart rhythm abnormalities.

Potassium is a mineral found in a wide variety of foods, such as bananas, tomatoes, and orange juice. Usually you can get enough of the potassium your body needs through the foods you eat.

Potassium moves in and out of muscle cells, creating electrical currents to make your muscles move. This is true for all muscles in your body, including those in your arms, legs, and torso. Low potassium levels in your body can cause profound muscle weakness, spasms, and cramps.

The heart is another muscle dependent upon potassium. When potassium levels become too low, or too high, abnormal electrical currents travel throughout the heart. The sudden discharge of these abnormal currents can cause the heart to pump irregularly, which may lead to a sustained spasm of the heart, followed by death.

You can lose potassium through vomiting and diarrhea. This potassium loss is normally replaced with many foods and beverages. But long periods of vomiting and diarrhea can result in dangerously low potassium levels, which can be checked with a simple blood test. Special potassium pills or liquids may be necessary to avoid a life-threatening abnormal heart rhythm.

High blood pressure can be associated with low potassium levels. Most water pills (or diuretics) used to treat high blood pressure, swelling, and heart failure can cause you to lose extra potassium in your urine. If you are taking a diuretic for any reason, you should have your blood potassium checked by your doctor on a regular basis. It may be important for you to take supplemental potassium pills or liquids, depending on your potassium level.

An overactive adrenal gland (located on top of each kidney) can cause a rare type of high blood pressure and profound potassium loss, requiring a special medication or surgical removal of part of the gland to maintain a normal potassium level.

Again, very high potassium levels can also cause heart-pumping irregularities, associated with certain medications, including the blood pressure pill known as the ACE inhibitor. Kidney disease can also cause high potassium levels. You should not take extra potassium pills without having your blood potassium levels monitored by your doctor.

In conclusion, if you experience muscle weakness and/or cramps, especially after diarrhea, vomiting, taking water pills, taking potassium supplements, taking the category of blood pressure pills called ACE inhibitors, or with a history of kidney disease, you should tell your doctor so he or she can monitor your potassium level. There are many causes of muscle cramps.

•

Dehydration

Tip 168:

If you are taking a steroid (including corti-
sone, prednisone, hydrocortisone, or methylpred-
nisolone) and you get sick with any illness, you
must be on the alert. Fatigue, muscle cramp or
weakness, and/or salt craving are your body's red
light warning signals of dehydration, and you
need emergency care. These symptoms can also
occur if you suddenly stop taking the steroids,
after taking them every day for a while, or if you
develop a disease in the adrenal glands.

The glands on top of your kidneys, the adrenal
glands, are small but very important for your body to
function normally. They produce steroids and other
essential hormones. One of their roles is to maintain a
balance of salt and water in your body.

Steroid-type medications can decrease the production of natural steroids by the adrenal glands. Usually the steroid medication substitutes for your natural steroid hormone. When you get sick, however, and your body needs even more of these hormones, these glands are so suppressed that you develop symptoms of dehydration from lack of steroids. Also, if you have been taking steroids for a while and you suddenly stop taking them, the adrenal glands may be so suppressed that you have none of these natural hormones immediately available and you become very ill. Muscle weakness, fatigue, muscle cramps, nausea, vomiting, and dehydration can develop very rapidly. Your blood pressure can drop to such low levels that death may result.

Rarely disease occurs in the adrenal glands, which directly affects their functioning. The pituitary gland, located under the brain, produces hormones that control the adrenal glands. When the pituitary gland is not working, the adrenal glands may also function improperly, causing the symptoms of dehydration.

Emergency medical treatment can save your life from dehydration when you do not have enough steroids in your body.

·

Fever

Tip 169:

Anytime your body temperature exceeds 99.8 degrees, you have a fever and something is causing it.

Having a fever does not mean feeling hot. It means an actual elevation of your body temperature, which is usually between 98.6 to 99.4 degrees. Normally your temperature is higher in the evening, but not over 99.4. (It begins to go down with total body inactivity during nighttime rest.) To allow for inaccuracies in taking your temperature, a good arbitrary level to set as being abnormal is 99.8 degrees. Therefore anytime it is above 99.8 degrees, you have a fever, and you need to know why.

Fever is an indication that your body is combating an illness such as a virus or bacterium infecting the body.

But cancer and various autoimmune diseases (where the body fights against itself) can also cause fever, and may be the only clue that illness is present. You should seek medical evaluation even if you have a persistently elevated temperature without an apparent cause. Early treatment of these illnesses often reduces the risk of serious complications. A fever over 103.5 degrees often represents a serious infection and should be evaluated immediately.

The pattern of rise and fall in body temperature may provide a clue to the cause of the fever. Therefore a chart monitoring temperature levels at various times may be helpful in diagnosing the problem. Also, when you have a fever, your temperature is often elevated in the evening but normal in the morning. You should never consider yourself well until your temperature has been normal for at least a twenty-four-hour period.

Tip 170:

Fever and continual drenching sweats at night suggest the presence of an infection such as tuberculosis or AIDS. Occasionally they occur with cancers, such as lymphomas and leukemia.

Long-term infections are notorious for causing fever at night. When fever occurs, and your body's temperature then returns to normal, drenching sweats result. The heat leaves the body with the sweat. This is part of the body's cooling mechanism. The sweats may be so profuse that you have to change your pajamas.

A common cause of night sweats is tuberculosis (TB),

whose other common symptoms include weight loss and a cough with or without bloody phlegm. TB is more likely to occur in people with weak immune systems (such as those with AIDS), those traveling to countries with a high TB infection rate, and those who have been exposed to TB patients. Drug abusers, patients who have had their stomachs surgically removed, and those who have been exposed to silica (the major component of sand, used in making glass) are also prime candidates for TB.

Night sweats are one of the early signs of an HIV infection, the virus that causes AIDS. They can occasionally be caused by cancer such as lymphoma.

Persistent night sweats and fever are red light warning signals to see your doctor for medical evaluation and treatment as soon as possible.

Medication

Tip 171:

If you stop taking a medication suddenly, you may develop serious complications. Therefore it is best to consult your doctor before stopping or decreasing the dosage of your medication.

Some medications cause serious problems if you suddenly stop taking them. Here are a few examples:

1. **High blood pressure pills.** If you suddenly stop taking certain blood pressure pills, not only will your blood pressure rise but in certain cases it will actually rise to such a high level that you could have a stroke. For example, stopping the drug Catapres (clonidine) may result in a very high "rebound" blood pressure. Other side effects may also occur. For example, suddenly stopping beta

blockers, in certain patients, can cause angina or a heart attack.

2. **Steroids.** Steroid pills may actually suppress your body's normal production of steroids. Therefore when you stop taking them, your body may react to the very low level of internally produced steroids. Your doctor should decrease the dosage slowly over time in order to allow the body to start producing the normal amount. (See Tip 168 for additional information on symptoms after stopping steroids.)

Since numerous medications can have a negative impact on your body if they are suddenly stopped, always consult your doctor before altering the prescribed directions for taking your medication.

•

Passing Out, Loss of Consciousness

Tip 172:

If someone has passed out, it is extremely important to know if they have had a seizure. Seizures can be recurrent and warrant specific treatment. They can also be a sign of an abnormality in the brain or an emergency life-threatening condition such as very low blood sugar or a serious mineral abnormality in the blood.

A seizure means there has been a sudden alteration of the electrical function of the brain. The brain generates electricity, which can be measured by a machine called an electroencephalogram (EEG). An EEG graphs out abnormal brain waves, indicating unusual electrical activity. A classic seizure involves a sudden loss of consciousness with jerking of the entire body, biting of the tongue, and urination, followed by a period of sleep before regaining consciousness.

If the electrical currents released by your brain are less intense and confined to a small area of the brain, a minor seizure will occur. The result of this minor seizure depends on the particular area of the brain involved. For example, you may just smack your lips or stare without knowing you are doing anything. Seizures occur in a wide variety of ways, since the brain has so many different functions. The spectrum includes experiencing a strange smell to experiencing an orgasm. The term *epilepsy* refers to seizures of unknown cause that often begin in childhood and continue throughout life.

The usual sign of an impending seizure is a special feeling called an "aura." The seizure—major or minor—in turn is followed by sleep or drowsiness, before normal behavior returns. This sequence of events—aura, altered consciousness with or without jerking, a period of sleep or altered awareness—separates seizures from fainting or other causes of sudden unconsciousness. The jerking phase of seizures usually lasts only a few minutes, while the postseizure sleeping period may last much longer. If the jerking phase does not stop after several minutes, or if it keeps recurring, the condition is life-threatening. Call an ambulance.

If you witness a person having a seizure who loses consciousness, turn him or her on his or her side, away from dangerous objects. Do not attempt to put anything in his or her mouth. Call for emergency care, unless the person is a known epileptic and you have been advised otherwise.

A common cause of a seizure in children is a high fever. As the brain matures into adulthood, it becomes less susceptible to this happening. (See Tip 190 for more information on seizures due to fevers in children.)

Seizures can result from a brain injury, brain tumor, or stroke. They can be caused by a life-threatening low or high blood sugar level, abnormal mineral levels in the blood, or a sudden loss of blood flow to your brain. These conditions need to be treated on an emergency basis. Therefore all first-time seizures require an immediate visit to the emergency room.

Seizures can also occur without an apparent cause. A normal adult with no previous history of seizures, no family history of epilepsy, and no current illness can suddenly have a major seizure. Medical tests may not show any cause. So what do you do? You often need to take medicine to control the seizures, since you cannot risk a recurrence while driving or in another potentially dangerous situation. If you have not had a seizure in many years, how long should you continue to use the seizure medicine? Only your doctor can make this judgment, based on your individual circumstances.

•

Temperature Change

Tip 173:

Prolonged exposure to cold can cause fatal body hypothermia.

The body's protective mechanisms maintain its temperature at around 98.6 degrees, which is necessary for its normal functions. Internal control mechanisms help maintain body temperature by routing blood away from the surface of the body and the extremities (arms and legs) and by shivering, to generate heat. If the body still cannot contain warmth, the body temperature drops and symptoms begin to appear. They are:

1. Confusion and forgetfulness
2. Sluggishness and fatigue
3. Incoordination
4. Slurred speech
5. Shivering (when shivering *stops,* the condition is getting worse)
6. Heart palpitations

Continued lowering of the body's temperature can produce coma and death.

If you encounter someone who is hypothermic:

1. Get the person to a warm room. Do not immerse them in a tub of hot water or place them in front of a heater or fireplace. The sudden exposure to excessive heat may worsen their condition.
2. Remove any wet clothing.
3. Cover the person with blankets.
4. Offer the person warm fluids, if they can drink. Do not give them an alcoholic beverage.
5. Seek out emergency medical assistance.

Tip 174:

Fatigue, dizziness, and/or headache are the first symptoms of heat exhaustion. Working or playing in the hot sun can be dangerous.

It is hard to tell when you are in danger of heat exhaustion. When you are active on a hot day, the body utilizes its cooling mechanism: sweating. The evaporation of sweat on the body's surface allows the body to get rid of heat. High humidity and the absence of a breeze can impair this mechanism. Individuals with fewer sweat glands are in greater danger of heat exhaustion. Senior citizens and young children are also more susceptible to heat exhaustion because the cooling mechanisms of their bodies are less effective.

Fluid loss and a rise in body temperature result in a serious derangement of body chemistry. Symptoms of heat exhaustion include:

1. Weakness, fatigue
2. Dizziness and/or headache
3. Incoordination and/or confusion
4. Muscle cramps
5. Vomiting, diarrhea
6. Low or no urine output
7. Pounding heartbeat

If you have any of the above symptoms, it is urgent that you do the following in order to avoid a heatstroke:

1. Move to the shade or indoors with air conditioning. Place a wet towel over your face, arms, and legs. Sit in front of a fan. Do not get in a bathtub of cold water.
2. Drink a lot of cold water.
3. Seek medical assistance. You may need to be given fluids intravenously or other therapy to cool down quickly.

The most important method of handling heat exhaustion is to prevent it. Take frequent breaks from exercise and exposure to heat. If you get tired, rest and cool off for a while. Drink a lot of water.

Tip 175:

Your thyroid gland does not have to be enlarged in order to be overactive or underactive. The variety of symptoms accompanying an overactive or underactive thyroid gland require early diagnosis and treatment to prevent serious complications.

The red light warning signals of an *overactive thyroid* are: intolerance to heat, a rapid and irregular pulse, tremors, fatigue, profuse sweating, increased appetite, etc.

The red light warning signals of an *underactive thyroid* are: cold intolerance, loss of memory, generalized body swelling (especially of the face), irregular and slow pulse, a high cholesterol level, etc.

The thyroid gland is located in the center of the base of the neck (see Figure 14). It serves as the body's thermostat, regulating the metabolic functions—that is to say, how quickly or slowly you burn up calories. An overactive thyroid promotes a rapid metabolic rate, while an underactive one slows it down.

The size of your thyroid gland has nothing to do with whether it is overactive or underactive. If the gland has not changed in size but is functioning abnormally, you may not seek treatment since the symptoms may develop gradually.

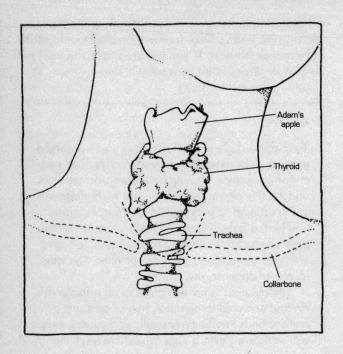

Figure 14. Thyroid Gland.

An overactive thyroid gland, producing excess thyroid hormone, causes intolerance to heat, a rapid and irregular pulse, tremors in the hands, profuse sweating, and sometimes heart failure.

An underactive thyroid produces an insufficient amount of thyroid hormone. The result is intolerance to cold, and you may feel cold all the time. Marked weakness and fatigue, loss of memory, paleness or a yellowish appearance, generalized body swelling (most prominent in the face), and a slow and sometimes irregular pulse are all characteristics of this disorder.

Both conditions can be associated with bulging eyes, fatigue, and double vision.

An overactive thyroid can cause dangerous heart rhythm abnormalities, while an underactive thyroid can result in a high cholesterol level. These and many other complications are a good reason to seek medical care as soon as possible when the symptoms creep up on you.

•

Weakness

Tip 176:

In senior citizens and diabetics a general sense of weakness without any chest pain may be the only warning sign of a heart attack.

Some heart attacks occur without any pain. A senior citizen or a diabetic may experience a general sense of weakness rather than chest pain.

The pain of a heart attack usually occurs in the center of the chest, under the breastbone or in the front-left breast area. The pain is most often a pressure sensation, like a heavy weight on the chest or a squeezing tightness. Profound weakness often accompanies the pain. A cold and clammy sweat may be present, with nausea and vomiting. In certain circumstances, however, a heart attack may occur in an entirely atypical manner.

If you are a senior citizen or diabetic, be aware that

profound weakness may be the only sign of a "silent" heart attack. Consult your physician immediately for an evaluation, which includes an EKG, blood tests of certain heart chemicals, and special X-rays of the heart, to determine if you are having a heart attack. Lifesaving treatments may be necessary.

Tip 177:

Muscle weakness, loss of memory, confusion, severe constipation, psychosis, and kidney stones are symptoms that may indicate an overactive parathyroid gland.

The parathyroid glands (there are usually four) are located in the front base of the neck near the thyroid gland. These small glands produce a hormone that controls the amount of calcium in your blood. If one of the glands develops a growth, or if the gland generally gets larger, the hormonal output is increased, causing the amount of calcium (stored primarily in the bones) to increase in the bloodstream.

A high level of calcium in the blood increases the risk of kidney stones. A high calcium level also causes muscle weakness, loss of memory, confusion, psychosis (loss of contact with reality), ulcer disease, and severe constipation. High levels of parathyroid hormone also cause loss of calcium from the bones, resulting in softening of the bones. The life-threatening consequences of high calcium include abnormal heart rhythms and severe dehydration.

Tumors or growths of the parathyroid glands are

rarely large enough to be felt by examining the neck, so you have to rely on appropriate blood studies to provide evidence that they are present.

Surgical removal of the diseased parathyroid gland is usually curative. Preservation of the remaining parathyroid glands is important since without them and the hormone they produce, the blood calcium level would drop too low, causing seizures and muscle spasms.

The symptoms of an overactive parathyroid gland can slowly creep up on you: muscle weakness, poor memory, confusion, constipation, and/or psychosis. If you develop these symptoms, notify your doctor for an evaluation as soon as possible.

Weight Loss

Tip 178:

If you have unexplained weight loss and/or loss of appetite, you may have a serious underlying medical illness.

How much weight loss is significant? If your body weight rarely changes, losing as little as five pounds could be significant. If your body weight varies eight to ten pounds from one season to another, you may be fine. But never ignore a weight loss of more than ten pounds. The more rapid the weight loss, the more likely it stems from a disease.

Body weight is determined by many different factors, including genetics, caloric intake, and physical activity. Caloric intake is the most important factor. Your body burns a certain number of calories per day, regardless of what you do. This is known as your basal metabolic rate (BMR). If you eat more calories than you burn, then you will gain weight, and if you eat fewer calories than you burn, you will lose weight.

Disease causes weight loss in numerous ways. Cancer releases substances into the system that can cause wasting of body tissues and/or loss of appetite. Diabetes results in an increase of sugar in the urine and therefore a loss in calories. An overactive thyroid gland increases the metabolic rate, therefore you burn more calories. Often you lose weight despite eating more. If you have an unexplained weight loss, you need medical evaluation as soon as possible.

Sometimes you may lose weight but your belly size actually increases. Liver and heart disease as well as cancer of the ovaries can cause fluid to accumulate in the belly cavity. Nonspecific symptoms like bloating, indigestion, heartburn, and changes in bowel habits may also occur with liver ailments and ovarian cancer. Therefore, if you lose weight, even though your waistline increases, it is important that you seek medical evaluation as soon as possible.

PART THREE

•

Pregnancy and Postpregnancy

Introduction

Preventive Measures to Increase the Chances of Delivering a Healthy Baby

A pregnant woman can take many preventive measures to increase the chances of delivering a healthy baby. Also, she should avoid certain medications, because the side effects can endanger the fetus.

It is important to be aware of past and existing illnesses as well as possible exposure to various diseases during pregnancy. For example, if the mother is exposed to hepatitis B or chicken pox, she and her baby can benefit from injections to reduce the risk of developing these ailments, which can be life-threatening. Unfortunately this book cannot address all the preventive measures that can increase the chances of delivering a healthy baby. We recommend that pregnant women be followed closely by their health care provider and seek out educational programs and literature addressing these issues. It is proven that early prenatal care reduces death rates for both mothers and infants.

Tip 179:

If you are pregnant and suffer from tenderness in the upper-right belly or upper-middle belly under the breastbone, a headache, blurred or double vision, dizziness, nosebleeds, and/or swelling or sudden weight gain, immediate medical evaluation is necessary since you may have very high blood pressure.

A condition called preeclampsia can cause severe high blood pressure, which can lead to seizures and coma (eclampsia). This condition appears during the last four months of pregnancy. Symptoms that may indicate preeclampsia include high blood pressure, plus upper-right or midbelly pain under the breastbone, nosebleeds, headache, dizziness, blurred vision, double vision, swelling, and/or sudden weight gain.

The exact cause of preeclampsia is not known. Changes in the body's blood pressure control mechanisms cause the blood vessels to narrow (constrict). The high blood pressure affects the kidneys, leading to significant weight gain and swelling. As the blood pressure rises to very high levels, you may also develop swelling in the brain and liver, leading to seizures and coma (eclampsia).

Seizures and coma are usually preventable when early treatment is instituted. If you develop the symptoms of preeclampsia, contact your doctor immediately.

Tip 180:

If you are pregnant with any of the following symptoms, seek immediate medical care: (1) severe belly pain, (2) leaking or breaking water, (3) decreased or absent fetal movements.

Certain infections during pregnancy can cause premature delivery. Thus if you have either of the following, contact your doctor immediately: (1) burning on urination or (2) a foul-smelling vaginal discharge.

Any of these symptoms may put your unborn baby at risk of developing serious health problems.

An emergency medical evaluation is needed for:

1. Severe belly pressure or pain. Such pain can be associated with internal bleeding in the uterus or rupture of the uterus at the site of the scar of a previous cesarean section.
2. Premature leaking or breaking of your water. This can cause a serious infection in the fetus. Also, in certain circumstances breaking water early can result in slippage and twisting of the umbilical cord, cutting off the oxygen supply and nutrition to the fetus.
3. Absence of fetal movement. If you do not feel the fetus move or feel a substantial change or decrease in fetal movement, this may indicate a life-threatening condition with your unborn baby.

To avoid premature delivery, immediately contact your doctor for:

4. Bladder infections. Such infections cause frequent urination, pain, and/or burning on urination. They can lead to a serious kidney infection, which can precipitate a premature delivery of the baby.
5. A foul or fishy-smelling vaginal discharge due to bacteria. This discharge may need treatment to avoid premature delivery of the baby.

Tip 181:

If you are pregnant but you have noted the reappearance of vaginal bleeding or cramping, it is important to check with your doctor immediately. This tip refers to the serious causes of vaginal bleeding or cramps seen during the first four months of pregnancy.

These causes include:

1. A threatened miscarriage, or a pregnancy that is failing. The embryo is likely to pass from the womb through the vagina. There is a possibility of severe bleeding.
2. An ectopic pregnancy. In this condition you are pregnant in your fallopian tube (pregnancy test may be positive or negative). An egg fertilized in the fallopian tube normally moves to the womb (uterus) and implants in the uterine wall, where it obtains nourishment and continues to grow. But if the egg

stays in the fallopian tube and continues to grow, it will rupture the tube. Severe life-threatening hemorrhage into the belly cavity may occur. You will not see the bleeding, although you may experience belly pain, weakness, a rapid pulse, dizziness, and a dark bloody vaginal discharge. Your pregnancy test may show changes. (Also see Tip 7 for more information on emergency internal bleeding.)

Both of these conditions require immediate treatment by a doctor. Therefore vaginal bleeding and/or cramping under these circumstances is a warning sign of a potentially life-threatening condition. These symptoms may also result from certain hormonal imbalances.

Tip 182:

Any bleeding, with or without belly cramps, during pregnancy deserves immediate medical evaluation. It may be a warning sign of a life-threatening hemorrhage. This tip refers to the serious causes of these red light warning signals after the fifth month of pregnancy.

Life-threatening causes of bleeding during the later stages of pregnancy are related to the location of the placenta or "afterbirth." Usually a fertilized egg situates itself inside the upper wall of the uterus or womb. As the embryo grows, it is connected to the placenta by the umbilical cord, which is attached to the uterine wall. The placenta is like a pancake, filled with lots of small blood vessels growing on the inside wall of the uterus.

If part of the placenta grows on the lower wall of the uterus, over the opening of the birth canal (called placenta previa), it is more likely to obstruct the baby's growth and delivery. It may also bleed at the spot where it is growing over this opening of the birth canal. Thus the unattached part of this pancakelike structure, filled with small blood vessels, will bleed into the uterine cavity (see Figure 15-A). When this occurs, you will see and feel blood coming out of your vagina. The bleeding is usually painless.

A normally placed placenta sometimes partially separates from the uterine wall and bleeds (called abruptio placentae—see Figure 15-B). This condition is usually accompanied by severe abdominal pain and/or strong uterine contractions.

In either case the baby can lose its blood supply, which deprives the baby of oxygen and nutrition. The baby's life is then in danger. Also, the mother's life may be in danger from the potential of massive internal bleeding. Emergency medical evaluation and treatment are necessary.

Tip 183:

If you think you are pregnant (missed periods and a positive pregnancy test), and experience severe nausea and vomiting, vaginal bleeding, and/or discharge of grapelike particles have it checked out. These symptoms may be due to a tumorlike growth in your womb. An early evaluation and therapeutic extraction of the mass can be lifesaving since you are in danger of hemorrhaging. About six percent of these growths are cancerous.

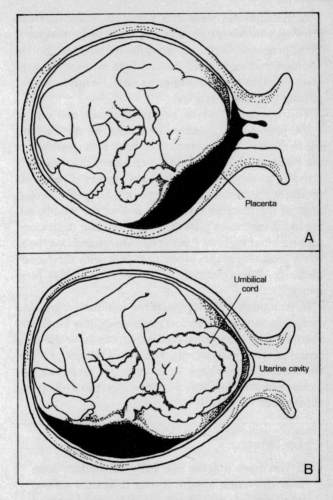

Figure 15. Vaginal Bleeding After the Fifth Month of Pregnancy.
A. Placenta previa
B. Abruptio placentae

A hydatidiform mole is a tumorlike mass that can grow in your womb so that you seem to be pregnant. Your pregnancy test will actually be positive. But in addition you experience the red light warning signals: severe nausea and vomiting, vaginal bleeding, and/or passing grapelike particles.

This condition, which occurs in about one out of 1,200 pregnancies, is caused by a defective egg implanting in the wall of the womb. The baby fails to grow, but the placenta (the pancakelike attachment that normally provides nourishment for the baby) grows rapidly and produces the hormones of pregnancy. Fingerlike projections of the placenta invade the wall of the womb, acting like a cancerous growth. They swell and degenerate, causing bleeding from the vagina. The projections themselves look like grapes when they pass with the bloody discharge. This condition is known as a "molar pregnancy."

If you think you are pregnant but have signs and symptoms suggesting a molar pregnancy, it is important that you seek emergency medical care to have the mass removed from your womb. You are in danger of a life-threatening hemorrhage. In addition, the fingerlike projections of the placenta can turn cancerous and spread throughout your body.

Tip 184:

If you have a fever and belly discomfort soon after delivering a baby, it may indicate a serious infection of the womb, which could spread rapidly. Heavy bleeding may also be a warning signal of a life-threatening hemorrhage.

You may already be home after delivering your baby when you develop a fever and belly pains. These symptoms may indicate an infection in your uterus (womb). This is dangerous because even a mild infection can spread rapidly throughout your body, since after delivery the internal lining of the uterus has many small blood vessels. Therefore, in this case, a mild infection can quickly become major. Immediate medical evaluation and treatment can be lifesaving.

If you are soaking blood through more than one pad (sanitary napkin) each hour, you are at risk of having a serious hemorrhage. Contact your health care provider immediately.

PART FOUR

•

Pediatrics: Body Part–Specific Conditions

by Joy Lawn, M.D.

Introduction
Childhood Conditions

Children are not just small adults. They suffer from many conditions that adults do not, and other conditions occur more commonly in children. It can be much more difficult to assess the health of a child, especially a younger child who cannot communicate clearly about his or her symptoms or cooperate fully with a doctor's examination.

Parents often fall into two groups: those who worry about everything concerning their child's health, and those who never seem nervous about anything. Unfortunately a parent may worry and consult the doctor frequently and still be worrying about the wrong things. This guide is intended to inform you about *what you do need to worry about in your child.*

This information is intended not to give you more to be nervous about but to direct you to important situations and conditions when you need medical help fast. This information should *reduce* your anxiety!

This chapter is not intended as an exhaustive guide on general pediatric conditions or as a first-aid guide. The conditions included have been chosen because:

1. The condition is a significant cause of childhood deaths or disability.
2. The condition is rare, but early diagnosis would make a big difference in the outcome of the child's survival.

How Do You Know When to Consult a Doctor Quickly?

Many parents with a sick child struggle with the decision to contact a doctor. Some see their child's doctor so often that the doctor's office feels like their living room! Yet even these parents may worry about an insignificant problem and not act quickly for a critical condition.

The following guidelines can help you know when you need to get your child to a doctor quickly.

I. Is Your Baby Really Ill?

Any baby under the age of three months should see a doctor on an emergency basis if they have any of the following:

A. Abnormal Temperature
1. Fever over 100.3 degrees. (Be sure that the baby is not overly wrapped or the room temperature too hot.) For children under 36 months of age, a rectal temperature is more accurate. (See Tip 221.)
2. Reduced temperature (less than 97 degrees), with no obvious cause

---

B. Sudden Onset of Feeding Difficulties
1. Intake of 50 percent or less of the normal amount of formula or breast milk intake

C. Change in Responsiveness
1. Sleepiness (being difficult to rouse), or sleeping much more than what is normal for them
2. Extreme irritability, crying inconsolably at the slightest stimulus

D. A significant sign or symptom as listed in II C or D

II. Is Your Child Really Ill?
Any child with a nonserious viral illness may be feverish and sleepy but should improve when the fever comes down. A child with any of the following should be seen on an emergency basis by a doctor:

A. High or Persistent Fever—levels and duration depend on symptoms, age, etc. Contact your doctor

B. Change in Responsiveness
1. Drowsiness
2. Extreme irritability (being difficult to calm)
3. Behavior that suggests the brain is not functioning properly, such as a failure to recognize people, seeing things not present, or fighting off attempts to help

C. The following symptoms:
1. Severe headache or recurrent headaches (see advice on headaches)

2. Convulsions (seizures)
3. Severe or bloody diarrhea
4. Severe belly pain
5. Markedly reduced urine production
6. Persistent vomiting, lasting more than 12 to 18 hours, or even 8 hours in the presence of diarrhea

D. Presenting with the following signs:
1. Very fast breathing (see table below)

Age	Breaths Per Minute
Under 3 months	Over 60
3 months to 2 years	Over 40
2 years to 10 years	Over 30
Over 10 years	Over 24

2. Slow, irregular breathing
3. Jaundice (yellow eyes or skin)
4. Cyanosis (blue color of mouth and lips)
5. Weakness of one part of the body
6. A change in vision or appearance of pupils
7. A bulging "soft spot" or fontanel on the head.
8. Floppy baby

Treatment of Rare but Potentially Correctable Life-Threatening Metabolic Disorders

Occasionally rare conditions which interfere with chemical processes within the body (known as metabolic disorders) occur and detection and early treatment may be lifesaving. For example, a lack of the substance carnitine is an infrequent cause of a life-threatening condition seen in young children in the emergency room. Once the more common causes of life-threatening conditions have been ruled out, the rare disorders should be considered. It is very important to inform your doctor of any clues of an underlying long-term ailment, such as poor weight gain, muscle weakness, or recurrent infections.

Prevention of Life-Threatening Conditions

In addition to being aware of red light warning signals, it is important to practice prevention. The death toll of children in developed countries could be cut dramatically if parents adhered to these recommendations:

- Breast-feed all babies for at least six months (although it is recommended that you breast-feed for at least one year if possible)
- Immunize all children (getting shots)
- Follow child safety regulations, and use car seats, bicycle helmets, etc.

•

Head

Headache

A Special Note on Assessment

Headache, one of the most common childhood complaints, has many simple causes. Yet it can also be an early warning signal for several very serious but less common conditions.

If the child has any of the specific symptoms listed in the descriptions below, call your doctor immediately. Even if you have a family history of migraines and you suspect your child has a migraine, this diagnosis should be established by a physician so that other conditions are not missed.

If the headache has any of the following characteristics, go to an emergency room:

1. **Timing:** It wakes the child from sleep or occurs early in the morning.
2. **Persistence:** It lasts over twenty-four hours consis-

tently, especially if worsening, or not responding to home treatment.

3. **Severity:** It is "the worst headache I've ever had" and does not respond to treatment.

4. **Associated with any of the following:**
   - a stiff neck
   - persistent vomiting
   - drowsiness or confusion
   - body weakness
   - unusual eye or limb movements
   - personality change
   - loss of previous skills such as walking

Tip 185:

A child with a headache, a stiff, painful neck, and fever should always be seen by a doctor immediately to exclude meningitis. Early diagnosis and treatment are critical. Children with meningitis often refuse to eat and want to be left alone.

Meningitis is an infection of the membranes covering the brain. It is most common in infants, who usually do not show specific signs (see Tip 221 for additional information on meningitis in infants). Bacterial meningitis is more serious than the viral type, and early diagnosis can dramatically reduce the chances of deafness, mental retardation, and death.

If your child has the above symptoms, especially associated with photophobia (sensitivity to light), he or she must be seen on an emergency basis by a doctor. In the early stages of meningitis, the child may not have a stiff neck.

Early treatment with intravenous antibiotics has a high cure rate (see Tip 3 for additional information on meningitis).

Tip 186:

Headaches in young children, especially when associated with vomiting or visual disturbances, should be taken very seriously and investigated in order to rule out a brain tumor.

Brain tumors are the most common type of childhood tumors, and in certain types of tumors, early diagnosis can make a big difference in survival. Increasing pressure on the brain causes headaches, usually in the morning, and these may be associated with vomiting and visual disturbances, most often double vision.

Other symptoms may include an unsteadiness during walking, slow growth in height, early puberty, or a personality change. Headaches can be caused by many nonserious conditions too, but it is important to have your child assessed and evaluated fully as soon as possible.

Tip 187:

Adolescents or young adults with headaches and visual changes may have a rare but treatable condition where the pressure on their brain is increased.

This condition, known as benign intracranial hypertension or pseudotumor cerebri, is more common in adolescent girls. It has many underlying causes, such as hormone imbalances, or a drug side effect (for example, following tetracycline or high doses of vitamin A). Frequently no specific cause can be found.

A spinal tap can show a very high pressure of the fluid on the brain. The condition is important because it may cause symptoms similar to a brain tumor but has a much better outcome. See your doctor as soon as possible for assessment and possible referral to a neurologist (brain specialist).

Tip 188:

If everyone in the whole household starts developing headaches, especially if associated with nausea and vomiting, it may be due to carbon monoxide poisoning. You must evacuate the house and seek urgent medical treatment.

A leaking gas furnace or pipe may result in carbon monoxide poisoning. Children are the first to be affected. Carbon monoxide poisoning can kill both children and adults quickly. If several people in the household develop headaches simultaneously, everyone should leave the house. Call the gas company, and get emergency medical attention. (See Tip 4 for additional information on carbon monoxide poisoning.)

Tip 189:

If your child has a head injury, is initially fine, and then becomes abnormally drowsy, vomits, or develops other symptoms within a few days, he or she may be experiencing bleeding inside the head. This is an emergency!

After a significant injury to the head, slow bleeding may start inside the top of the head, and the child may gradually get drowsy due to increasing pressure within the head. If your child injures his or her head and initially seems fine, observe the child closely for at least the next two or three days. This includes waking the child every couple of hours to make sure he or she has not lost consciousness. Go to the hospital emergency room or call an ambulance (911 in some locations) if your child gets more drowsy, experiences weakness or jerking in one side of the body, develops double vision, or exhibits any other major changes (see Tip 9 for more information on head injuries).

Tip 190:

If your child has a fever and starts convulsing, the convulsions (seizures) will normally be over within a few minutes, and it is important that you know how to react in this situation.

Children between the ages of six months and six years with a high fever are at risk of convulsing. This condition is known as a febrile convulsion. It is more common in children who have a relative who has had febrile seizures. The seizure usually occurs early in an illness, during the first spike of fever. In fact, it may even be the first sign of a febrile illness.

It is upsetting to see your child convulsing. A simple febrile seizure lasts less than ten minutes, and a large proportion last less than five minutes, so try to be calm and do the following:

1. **Lay your child on a soft surface** (usually the floor) on their side. Do not try to restrain him or her.
2. **Remove any vomit or saliva from his or her mouth.** Do not try to insert a spoon into the mouth—it will do more harm than good. Do not put your fingers in the child's mouth, or you may lose a finger!
3. **Time the seizure and if it lasts longer than five minutes or recurs within twenty-four hours, or affects only one side of the body, call an ambulance (911 in most locations).** If it stops before five minutes, call your pediatrician **immediately** for advice. In a first episode for a child under 18 months, more evaluation will be needed to rule out causes such as meningitis. In all cases notify your doctor about the seizure.
4. **Immediately after the seizure remove the child's clothes.** Sponge the child with lukewarm water if the temperature is over 103 degrees. **Do not let the child get chilled, otherwise the temperature will go back up.**
5. **Do not give the child anything to eat or drink immediately after the seizure until he or she is able to respond to you. Then give an antifever medi-**

cine other than aspirin (ibuprofen or an acetaminophen, such as Tylenol).

If your child has had a febrile convulsion, he or she
has an approximately 33 percent chance of having
another seizure within the year following the episode.
The risk continues to decrease over time. Less than 2
percent of children with simple febrile seizures will go
on to develop epilepsy. For a child with a simple febrile
convulsion, there is no association with learning difficulties later.

Tip 191:

**Convulsions in a baby can be very subtle. If your
baby has unusual rhythmic movements, especially in the face or limbs, call a doctor.**

In adults the most common type of convulsion is a
generalized one, where the whole body shakes violently
and the person is unaware of their surroundings. In
babies, especially in the first month of life, these seizures
are more subtle. A baby may "cycle" a leg repetitively
for a minute, which may be the only obvious sign of a
convulsion.

If your baby has *repeated* unusual rhythmic movements, especially in the context of other problems such
as feeding difficulties or a complicated delivery, keep a
record and description of these episodes, and consult
your doctor as soon as possible. Some jerking movements of babies, especially when asleep, may be normal.

Psychological Problems

Tip 192:

If you suspect that your child or adolescent may be depressed, seek urgent appropriate help because suicide is the second most common cause of death among teenagers.

Depression can happen in even the most loving home. Even if it is precipitated by a personal crisis, it is usually caused by a chemical imbalance. A family predisposition may also be an influence. Children and teenagers with depression are often labeled as "difficult" or "moody" rather than given appropriate help. The stigma of depression can also cause people to avoid seeking help—a delay that can have tragic results.

Clinical depression is a prolonged, persistent disturbance of moods, often having associated physical symptoms. The warning signs may include:

1. Persistent sadness and complaints, with a negative self-image
2. Lack of interest in favorite activities and food
3. Withdrawal from family and friends, at times with hostility
4. Worsening school performance
5. Anxiety about simple tasks and events
6. Sleep disturbances, either insomnia or hypersomnia (long periods of sleep)
7. Appetite changes: loss of appetite or overeating
8. Multiple physical complaints: aches and pains everywhere
9. Hinting at suicide or giving away prized possessions

If your child exhibits any of the above symptoms, get them assessed and treated before they injure themselves seriously.

Risk Factors for Suicides

- Male (although more girls attempt suicide, more boys actually succeed)
- Alcohol or drug abuse
- A gun in the house (firearms are used the most to commit suicide in America)
- A previous suicide attempt
- A recent suicide in your area
- A bereavement experience: a death, a divorce, a failed exam, rejection by friends, and the like

With counseling and medication (if appropriate), your child can go on to live a full and normal life.

Tip 193:

Anorexia and bulimia are not just social problems. They are dangerous, life-threatening conditions needing expert treatment as soon as possible. Overeating and obesity can also be serious health hazards.

Anorexia is common in preadolescent and adolescent girls. The individual has an overpowering fear of being fat, accompanied by behavior intended to result in weight loss, such as not eating, excessive exercise, etc. Bulimia tends to occur in older adolescents or adults and is associated with binge eating and purging (self-induced vomiting or use of laxatives). Bulimics are at additional risk of dying because self-induced vomiting and purging with laxatives often cause dangerous imbalances in the blood.

An affected teenager may:

- Avoid eating with the family and eat very little
- Use laxatives and induce vomiting
- Exercise excessively
- Wear shapeless clothes
- Have irregular menstrual periods
- Develop fine, downy hairs on the face and trunk

The earlier a diagnosis is made and professional help obtained, the better chance that your daughter will have a normal adult life. Lead her by positive example with good eating habits!

•

Eyes

Tip 194:

Two red light warning signals that may indicate a tumor in the back of the eye are:

1. "Unparallel" eyes—one eye looks straight ahead and the other looks in a different direction (this may be normal under four months of age, but still consult your pediatrician).
2. One pupil appears white or consistently different from the other pupil.

If your child has either of these, it is important to have him or her assessed by an ophthalmologist (eye specialist).

Tumors of the retina (in the back of the eye) usually occur in the first two years of life and are more common in children with a family history of this condition. There is usually no pain with this tumor, which is known as a retinoblastoma.

Over 90 percent of the children with this eye tumor can be cured with early diagnosis. A rapid diagnosis and treatment increase the chances of preserving sight in the affected eye and saving the child's life. Genetic evaluation of the child and family should be undertaken, because some of these cases are hereditary.

Throat

Tip 195:

Chronic hoarseness may be the first sign of warts on the vocal cords, so the child should be assessed. If the warts grow large, they can obstruct breathing.

Children are often hoarse for a short period after a cold—or too much shouting! If your child (especially a child under five) has hoarseness repeatedly for more than two weeks, however, you should take the child to the doctor to ensure that there are no growths on their vocal cords that could compromise breathing.

Tip 196:

If a child has become suddenly ill and has a throat that is so sore that he or she cannot swallow any liquids, especially with drooling, difficulty talking or breathing, take your child to the emergency room immediately (or call an ambulance, which is 911 in many areas). Swelling, which may have occurred with the infection, could be completely blocking the child's throat.

Children may not want to eat or drink when sick. But when given a pain or fever reducer, they can usually be convinced to take small amounts of cool liquids. If your child refuses to take any liquids, even after being given the correct dose of an over-the-counter pain medicine and, especially if they cannot swallow their own saliva and are drooling, a doctor should see the child on an emergency basis. Swelling may have occurred in the throat due to infection, which could be blocking the child's airway. If your child appears very ill, has difficulty swallowing, talking or breathing, he or she needs to be taken to the hospital.

Arms, Hands, Fingers, and Nails

Tip 197:

An infant with swollen, tender fingers or toes may be showing the first signs of sickle cell disease. Early diagnosis and treatment reduce the risk of dying very young.

Sickle cell disease is an inherited disorder common in the African and African American community (one in 500). It also occurs in people from Asia, the Mediterranean, and South America. The condition affects the shape of red blood cells and causes anemia (a low red blood cell count). The abnormal red blood cells block the blood vessels, resulting in pain and a high risk of infection, especially from certain bacteria. Twenty-five percent of children with this condition will die before they reach the age of five, yet with appropriate treatment and education, many sickle cell sufferers will survive to their fifties or older.

The typical first signs in an infant are swollen, tender, red, shiny fingers or toes. The signs may last for several days. The fingers and toes are very painful, and the infant may be distressed. An older, school-age child or adult tends to have pain in the arms, legs, and belly.

The diagnosis can be made from a simple blood test. Seek medical advice on how to deal with the various problems relating to this ailment. If younger children with sickle cell disease take certain antibiotics regularly, they will often reduce the risk of developing life-threatening infections.

Back

Tip 198:

If your teenager's back and ribs appear asymmetrical (especially when bending over to touch his or her toes), he or she may be developing a curved spine. It can get worse rapidly, causing serious problems.

Progressive curvature of the spine occurs more commonly in adolescent girls. Rapid worsening of the curvature results in severe deformity and breathing difficulties. Early treatment may prevent progression; occasionally surgery is needed.

If you suspect this condition, look at your child's back from behind while she is touching her toes. Note if the ribs on one side (in 80 percent it will be on the right side) form a hump (see Figure 16). The shoulder blade may also appear to protrude on the same side. If you suspect your child has this condition, seek medical evaluation and treatment early.

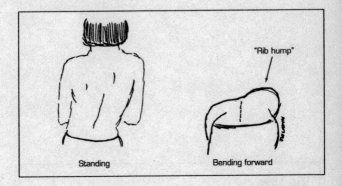

Figure 16. Girl with Scoliosis.

Chest

Tip 199:

A child who suddenly develops a harsh noisy sound when breathing in (called stridor) should be seen immediately in an emergency room.

Sudden onset of stridor is usually associated with difficulty in breathing. The most common cause of a sudden onset of stridor used to be an infection of the epiglottis (a "hinged" flap over the windpipe, which stops food from entering the lungs when you swallow). This is very rare now (thanks to HIB immunization), which protects children from the germ causing this problem. This condition is life-threatening and the child needs to be seen in an emergency room immediately. Do not administer first aid for choking because this could make the condition worse.

Croup and inhaled objects are the remaining common

serious causes of stridor. If you suspect an infant has inhaled an object (such as a little toy, peanut, coin, or battery) and if he or she has a sudden onset of difficulty breathing, immediately administer first aid. (See Appendix A for basic instructions.)

Croup is a viral infection around the voice box that causes a typical barklike cough. It is usually gradual in onset and not serious, but it is still important to notify your pediatrician. However, if a younger child with this ailment develops noisy breathing, it may be life-threatening. Keep the child as calm as possible (agitation worsens the condition), and get the child to an emergency room immediately. Do not administer first aid for choking because this could make the condition worse.

Tip 200:

If your child has recurrent wheezing, especially when he or she gets a cold, or a recurrent night-time cough, he or she may have asthma and should be assessed and started on appropriate treatment.

Asthma is an allergic condition. Certain triggers cause the small "air pipes" in the lungs to become inflamed, making breathing more difficult and causing the individual to wheeze, cough, and, if severe, even struggle for breath. The most frequent trigger in young children is a cold. In the school-age child, exercise and allergens (like cats, dogs, house dust, mites, certain foods) are more of a problem.

Asthma is increasingly common, and many cases occur in families with no previous history of allergy. Sometimes the child may simply have a recurrent night-time cough, and the diagnosis of asthma may be delayed, which can have serious consequences. Asthma is a variable condition, and most children have mild disorders that are easily treatable usually, with inhaled daily preventative medicine. Many will "grow out of it." Some children, however, will get severe life-threatening attacks. So have your child assessed by a doctor as soon as possible for appropriate treatment, and learn to avoid the "triggers" of his or her particular asthma attack (see Tip 49 for more information on an asthma attack).

Tip 201:

If you know your child has asthma—that is, struggling to breathe, difficulty speaking, possibly turning blue—you should be able to recognize a severe attack and know how to react immediately. You should also learn what triggers severe attacks of asthma for your child and try to avoid these triggers.

Five to six million children in the United States have asthma. A severe attack can be rapidly life-threatening in a child, whereas a mild attack may be managed carefully with home treatment with inhaled medication (using a nebulizer or a metered dose inhaler with a spacer), in consultation with your physician. You need to be able to recognize a severe attack. The child will struggle to breathe, be unable to speak easily, or to walk across the room, and possibly even turn blue. The loudness of the wheeze is irrelevant, and in fact a "silent chest" is more serious. Call for an ambulance (911 in many locations), and while you are waiting, start your child on inhaled medication, if you have it (see Tip 49 for more information on an asthma attack).

Belly

Tip 202:

If you have a child between the ages of two and six, you should observe his or her belly every few weeks for any masses. Early diagnosis and treatment of a mass observed or felt in the belly will increase the chances of survival if he or she has kidney cancer.

Wilms' tumor of the kidney occurs mainly in the two-to-six-year age group, with a peak at the age of three. At the time of diagnosis, most children seem well and are simply found to have a large mass in the belly area. Often the mass has become surprisingly large before the parents even notice its presence. Twenty-five percent of children with Wilms' tumor will also have a small amount of blood in the urine, which is often not visible and shows up only in testing the urine.

Children with any of the following are at increased risk of Wilms' tumor:

1. Abnormal kidney shape or structure (like horse-shoe kidney) from birth
2. Genital abnormalities (like hypospadias)
3. A family history of Wilms' tumor
4. Certain syndromes, especially if one side of the child's body is bigger than the other (hemihypertrophy)
5. No iris in the eye
6. Abnormalities of chromosome II (detected by a blood test)

Children with any of these risk factors should be checked regularly by a doctor to exclude a kidney tumor. Early diagnosis will result in cure rates around 90 percent.

Urine

Usually after bloody diarrhea typically caused by the bacteria *E. coli* 0157, or more rarely after a respiratory infection, a child may suddenly develop temporary kidney failure and severe anemia. This is called hemolytic-uremic syndrome and is more common in children under the age of three. The child will have markedly reduced urine output and may be drowsy, irritable, and pale. Needlepoint red spots on the skin can be another sign of this illness. Emergency medical therapy improves the chance for survival and lowers the risk of long-term kidney problems.

Tip 204:

If your child is experiencing frequent, sometimes painful, urination with a strong smell and mild fever, he or she may have a urinary tract infection. The signs in a child are subtle, so it is important to be aware of them and take this condition seriously. Recurrent, untreated urinary tract infections in young children are the most common cause of kidney failure, which may result in premature death as an adult.

Urinary tract infections (UTIs) in infants and young children can be extremely difficult to diagnose because the symptoms are usually nonspecific: mild fever, more frequent urination (sometimes with pain), or urine that smells particularly strong. The difficulty in diagnosis is compounded by the struggle to get a clean sample of urine from a small child.

If your child has a fever with no other obvious cause (such as a cold or ear infection), you should have his or her urine checked by a doctor as soon as possible. If your preschool child has had a proven UTI, he or she should be thoroughly checked, in order to exclude a problem where the urine refluxes up into the kidney from the bladder. A child who has this reflux problem is at higher risk of damaging the kidneys and needs to be carefully supervised and treated. A delay in diagnosis and treatment can result in permanent kidney damage and high blood pressure later in life. (See also Tip 122.)

Tip 205:

If your child is drinking much more than normal, passing a lot of urine, and losing weight, you should get him or her tested to exclude diabetes mellitus. Early diagnosis and treatment can improve overall long-term health.

Many children with diabetes mellitus are not diagnosed until they go into a coma and develop a life-threatening condition called ketoacidosis. In retrospect most parents of newly diagnosed diabetics realize that their child has not been "right" for weeks or even months, often displaying symptoms of weight loss, low energy, and excessive thirst.

Parents who notice these symptoms in their child should take the child for a checkup as soon as possible, especially if there is a family history of diabetes. Any child who has previously been dry by night but then starts bed-wetting should have a urine check for diabetes. If a diagnosis of diabetes is made, careful control of the child's blood sugar (with diet and insulin injections) can decrease the risk of the later complications of diabetes.

Bowel Movement

Tip 206:

If your baby has suffered from chronic constipation since birth, he or she may have an abnormality in the nerve supply to the large bowel or a defective anus. This condition requires surgery to prevent bowel obstruction and life-threatening inflammation or perforation of the bowel.

Hirschsprung's disease is a condition in which the nerve supply to the large bowel is abnormal. Boys are affected about five times more commonly than girls, and the disease is more frequent in children with Down's syndrome. The symptoms depend on the length of bowel affected, which varies from a few centimeters near the anus to the whole length of the large bowel.

If only a short segment of bowel is involved, the diagnosis may be delayed. Any baby who does not pass a stool in the first forty-eight hours of life and does not have an obvious bowel or anal abnormality should be investigated for this condition. Any child who has been constipated since birth should also be investigated. Constipation while potty-training, in a toddler with previously normal bowel habits, is usually normal. If a diagnosis is not made, the child's bowel may become blocked and inflamed and may burst (perforate).

Tip 207:

If your infant is crying abnormally, pulling up his or her knees, or passing stools that look like jelly, he or she needs to be seen immediately at an emergency room.

Babies may get a condition in their bowels (called intussusception) where one portion of the bowel telescopes into the next and gets stuck. This blocks the bowel and cuts off the blood supply to that portion of bowel. If the condition is not reversed rapidly, the bowel will die, and the infant will become very ill.

It may be difficult to differentiate a baby with colic (spasmodic pain in the abdomen) from one with intussusception. Initially the baby with intussusception may cry intermittently and then all the time. A sausage-shaped lump may be felt in the belly. The baby may pass jellylike stools. If the condition is diagnosed early, it can often be cured by a special enema, avoiding the need for surgery. This should always be done by an experienced doctor. This is an emergency. Get the child to an emergency room immediately.

Tip 208:

If a child or infant has more than a very small amount of blood in his or her stools during an episode of diarrhea, it increases the chance that the illness is a serious one and will require immediate medical attention.

Older children may flush the toilet without observing the nature of a diarrhea stool. They should be asked to look at the stool and show it to an adult if it is abnormal. With the emergence of *E. coli* as a very dangerous germ, it has become important that parents watch diarrhea carefully (see Tip 209 for more emergency information on diarrhea in babies and children). Large numbers of stools, severe cramping with diarrhea, and blood in the stools should cause parents to seek immediate medical attention.

Remember, when observing the stool, that if the child drinks red liquids, the stool may have a red color.

Tip 209:

In a baby or child who has diarrhea, with or without vomiting, dehydration due to excessive loss of fluid should be avoided—it can be life-threatening.

Diarrhea (the passage of frequent, runny stools) and vomiting are both common problems in babies and infants. Dehydration can occur rapidly, especially if the infant also has fever.

If your child has diarrhea and/or vomiting and any of the following, you should get him or her to the emergency room.

1. Frequent loose stools (more than four in four hours) or vomiting (more than three in four hours), at under three months of age
2. Signs of dehydration:
   a. Excessive drowsiness or irritability, or limpness
   b. Sunken eyes and sunken fontanel (soft spot on the head)
   c. Loose, dry skin
   d. Dry mouth and tongue
   e. Very little, dark-colored urine (less than three wet diapers in twenty-four hours)
3. Associated fever over 101 degrees, which does not respond to simple treatment
4. Persistent belly pain
5. Blood in the stools
6. Very forceful, recurrent vomiting (projectile), in a baby; green or bloody vomit

In children over six months, dehydration should be avoided by giving oral rehydration solutions such as Pedialyte, Infantlyte, or Rehydralyte. These solutions should not be used in babies younger than six months without the advice of a physician. They are best when given in small volumes at frequent intervals, and they are very effective even if your child is still vomiting occasionally. Sometimes you may have to give as little as a teaspoon at a time.

Viruses are the most common cause of diarrhea in children. Babies who are exclusively breast-fed to six months of age very rarely get significant diarrhea. Eating undercooked ground beef and unwashed vegetables increases the risk for the dangerous *E. coli* diarrhea.

Genitalia

Tip 210:

If your child develops signs of puberty too early, such as pubic and axillary hair, breast enlargement, increasing genitalia size, he or she should be evaluated, as it can be due to a hormone problem or a tumor in the brain or an adrenal gland.

Signs of puberty, such as pubic hair, hair in the armpits, breast development, and increasing genitalia size, are considered abnormal when developed under the age of eight years in girl and ten in boys. Precocious or early puberty has many nonserious causes, but it is important to rule out tumors of the brain or adrenal gland (located on top of the kidney) and hormonal problems. Take your child to the doctor for assessment and possible investigation. Early diagnosis of a tumor may be lifesaving.

Legs

Tip 211:

If your son learned to walk late and has difficulty standing up from a sitting position or going upstairs, you must take him to a doctor to be sure it is not a muscular dystrophy such as Duchenne's.

The most common muscular dystrophy occurs only in boys (about one in every 2,500 male births). Many cases are in families with no previous history of this condition.

The boy is usually slow to learn to walk (over 18 months old) and has difficulty climbing stairs or getting into the car. He may get up from sitting on the floor by climbing up his legs. He may waddle as he walks and tends to fall a lot. His calf muscles may look bigger than normal. Thirty percent of boys with this condition will also have associated learning difficulties. Treatment is supportive rather than curative, but early diagnosis allows for genetic counseling about future pregnancies.

Tip 212:

If your child starts complaining of significant, persistent pain in the bones, especially around the knee, he or she should be seen by a doctor to exclude cancer of the blood or of the bone. Most bone pains in children are not serious.

Acute lymphoblastic leukemia is a cancer of the blood and is the most common childhood cancer, occurring especially in two-to-six-year-olds. Two-thirds of children with this cancer complain first of bone pain, often around the knee. A preverbal child may simply cry a lot and want to be carried much more frequently. Sometimes the diagnosis is delayed because no one thinks of cancer. This cancer has a 90 percent cure rate, especially if diagnosed early.

The most common childhood bone tumors occur in boys around the time of puberty. Early diagnosis is important because once the cancer has spread elsewhere in the body, the prognosis gets much worse.

Obviously lots of simple causes for leg pains in active children are not worth worrying about. But if the pain is severe and constant, you should take your child to the doctor to rule out serious causes.

Skin and Hair

Tip 213:

A child with high fever (over 101 degrees), often with nausea and vomiting, and a red or purple flat blotchy rash that does not disappear when pressed could have a serious bacterial blood infection (meningococcosis) and should be seen immediately in the emergency room.

Fever and rash in a child have many causes. The majority are viral, such as chicken pox, measles, etc. In a normal child they are not usually life-threatening. But if your child suddenly develops a fever with a rash that is red and flat, typically most obviously over the buttocks, *This Is an Emergency!!* Even a one-hour delay could affect your child's chances of survival. Get your child to an emergency room.

One cause is a bacterium called meningococcus,

which produces a serious infection in the blood that progresses rapidly. It often responds well to early treatment with intravenous antibiotics. Other emergency medical conditions including inflammation of blood vessels after a viral infection can also cause these symptoms.

The same rash with no fever in a well child could be due to a reduced number of platelets in the blood, which puts the child at risk of severe bleeding, such as a brain hemorrhage.

Tip 214:

A red, flat birthmark covering approximately one-third of a child's face on one side may be associated with serious underlying brain abnormalities. The child should be thoroughly investigated by a physician.

In Sturge-Weber syndrome the child has a red, flat birthmark covering one third of the face. There is an underlying abnormality, usually in the back area of the brain, on the same side. It may result in epilepsy, mental retardation, and a stroke, affecting the opposite side of the body. Expert neurological (nerve) and ophthalmological (eye) assessment and care are needed to prevent or treat possible complications associated with this condition. The condition is not thought to be inherited.

Tip 215:

If your child has developed freckling and increased coloration of the skin around his or her mouth or anus, he or she may have a condition called Peutz-Jeghers syndrome. He or she may also have multiple polyps (fingerlike growths) throughout the bowel, which may bleed, causing anemia (a low blood count) or bowel blockage.

Peutz-Jeghers syndrome, a genetic condition, has a 50 percent chance of inheritance. The affected person has increased pigmentation and freckling around the mouth and often around the anus as well. This pigmentation can be a red light warning signal of polyps in the wall of the gut. The polyps often bleed, resulting in anemia, and may also cause intussusception (where one part of the gut telescopes into the next). Cancerous change is usually not thought to occur in these polyps. The child (or adult) should be assessed thoroughly by a gastroenterologist (stomach/intestine specialist). (See Tip 148 for more information on this disorder.)

> **Tip 216:**
>
> Does your child have five or more flat brown birthmarks (each more than 1.5 centimeters in diameter)? If so, he or she should be examined by an expert to exclude neurofibromatosis, an important inheritable condition that may be associated with learning disabilities, epilepsy and a high risk of malignant tumors.

Neurofibromatosis, an inherited condition, is not uncommon, with an incidence of one per 2,500 of the population. It is very variable in its manifestations. A child who has one or more of the following should be assessed by an expert:

1. Five or more "café au lait" spots (light brown flat moles) on the skin (each measuring over 1.5 centimeters in diameter). They are most commonly found on the trunk of the body, and are usually not present at birth but appear in the first two decades of life.
2. Freckling in the armpits.
3. Plexiform neurofibroma, a lumpy overgrowth of parts of peripheral nerves, most common on the jaw and eyelids.
4. Fibromas, or small, pink, nonpainful lumpy growths on the skin that do not occur until puberty.
5. Speckling on the surface of the eye.

Adults may have neurofibromatosis but be unaware of it. Affected children may present with neurological problems during infancy, such as epilepsy, attention deficit disorder, and mental retardation. Those affected are at high risk of developing tumors of the nerve to the eye, the main nerve to the ear, and brain tumors. A precise diagnosis is especially important for genetic consulting of the family.

Tip 217:

In a young, very irritable child with fever, red eyes and mouth (redder than normal), a rash, peeling skin on the hands and feet, and/or enlarged neck glands, expert assessment is needed to rule out Kawasaki's disease. Early diagnosis and appropriate treatment are essential to prevent life-threatening heart problems.

Kawasaki's disease may initially resemble many other childhood illnesses, but it is important to make the diagnosis and treat the condition as early as possible. Treatment usually includes gamma-globulin and low-dose aspirin to prevent the formation of aneurysms (outpouching) in the arteries supplying blood to the heart muscle, which may cause a "heart attack" in young children. The condition is more common in Japanese children.

The typical case is a child under five with a sudden onset of a high fever (over 104 degrees) lasting for several days, and at least four of the following features:

1. Light sensitivity and red eyes
2. Mouth and lips are more red than normal

3. Changes in hands and feet (initially swollen, then red and peeling)
4. Rash (often more severe in the anal area)
5. Swollen glands in the neck

See your doctor as soon as possible. Early treatment with intravenous gamma-globulin is proven to protect against its life-threatening aspects.

Tip 218:

If your baby is jaundiced (has a yellow hue to the skin and/or eyes) during the first week of life, he or she needs to be assessed immediately by a doctor in order to determine if there is risk of life-threatening complications from high levels of the substance bilirubin.

Jaundice in the first week of life may be very serious. If the bilirubin (the substance that causes the jaundice) reaches high levels, it can cross into the brain, causing brain damage or even death. Mild jaundice is very common, affecting 80 percent of premature babies and 60 percent of regular term babies, and is not serious. But several causes of jaundice may result in a seriously high level of bilirubin.

A common cause of severe jaundice is an incompatibility between the mother's blood type and the baby's blood type. An inherited red blood cell disorder, including G6P deficiency and sickle cell disease, can also cause severe jaundice. In these cases red blood cells are destroyed, and the bilirubin is released into the bloodstream causing the yellow coloring. Both of these conditions occur much more commonly in Asians and African Americans than in Caucasians. Unfortunately, despite their high risk, jaundice is harder to detect in these babies due to skin coloring. Their jaundice is more clearly seen in the whites of the eyes or in the gums than in the skin.

Jaundice during the first weeks of life may also be caused by an extremely serious bacterial infection in the blood.

During the first weeks of life, babies have their eyes closed most of the time, so parents have to make a conscious effort to look carefully every day for the first week. Gently open the eyes and mouth to check for signs.

If there is no underlying illness, mild jaundice requires no treatment. Moderate jaundice can be treated easily by putting the baby under a special blue light, thus preventing the jaundice from becoming more serious. Severe jaundice may require an exchange blood transfusion, which is a major procedure.

If your baby has these red light warning signals, see your doctor as soon as possible.

Tip 219:

A child with an inherited disorder of sparse hair, fragile nails, pointed teeth, and dry skin may be unable to control his or her temperature and could die from extreme heat or from a high temperature.

Several conditions, collectively called the ectodermal dysplasias, involve inherited abnormalities of hair, nails, teeth, and skin. Children affected by these conditions will have dry, sparse hair, fragile, cracked fingernails, and dry skin. Some also have pointed teeth.

Since the ability to sweat may be impaired, the child may be unable to regulate his or her temperature and become dangerously hot (hyperthermic). You must take specific measures to keep your child from overheating. A child with this condition should be assessed by a skin specialist (dermatologist).

•

Allergic Reactions

Tip 220:

In susceptible individuals a severe allergic reaction affecting the entire body (anaphylactic shock) may follow an insect sting or the ingestion of certain medications or foods. The red light warning signals include: sudden swelling of the lips and tongue, difficulty breathing, weakness, and a feeling of faintness. Immediate emergency care is required to prevent death.

Certain individuals, especially those who are more prone to allergies or who have a family member who has had a life-threatening reaction to an allergen (anaphylactic shock), may have a severe reaction to certain substances.

The most common causes are:

1. Insect bites
2. Medications, especially the penicillin family
3. Foods such as peanuts, shellfish, and strawberries

The individual may feel a burning of the lips and, within minutes, have a puffy face and neck and be struggling to breathe. They may complain of belly pain, have bloody diarrhea, and develop a blotchy, red raised rash. *Call an ambulance immediately.* (Or dial 911 in most locations.)

If you or your child has had a reaction like this one before, always carry an epinephrine injection kit (e.g., EpiPen) with you, and know how to use it. For an older child, teach him or her how to self-administer the injection. Get an identity bracelet, clearly showing the medical details of the problem and necessary treatment. An allergist should also be consulted. The allergist may be able to reduce the severity of these reactions. (See Tip 160 for more information on allergies.)

Fever

Get the baby to the doctor or an emergency room immediately in the following situations:

1) The child is under 3 months of age with a fever over 100.3 degrees measured rectally;
2) The child is between 3 and 15 months of age with a fever of 100.3 degrees or greater, and is either irritable, difficult to arouse, or not drinking;
3) The child's fever comes down, but the child is still irritable, difficult to arouse and/or not drinking liquids.

4) The child's fever is over 103.6 degrees.

   Also, call your doctor if the child has had a fever over 100.3 degrees for twenty-four hours or more.

Babies get meningitis (infection of the membranes covering the brain) more commonly than adults do, yet they obviously cannot complain of a headache. Before the baby's soft spot on top of his or her head is closed, the infant is less likely to show the classic physical signs that doctors test for, such as a stiff neck. About 25 percent of babies with meningitis will have a bulging soft spot. Under the circumstances just listed, it is very important to get your baby to an emergency room immediately because meningitis is a life-threatening condition. Do not overwrap your baby, as this may raise the temperature further. The doctor needs to determine if meningitis is the diagnosis. Urgent treatment is essential.

•

Miscellaneous

Tip 222:

The loss of a number of basic skills, such as
walking and talking clearly, is known as developmental regression. It has a number of serious
causes, and the child should be thoroughly evaluated.

Occasionally when a child has been ill or has had
a major emotional upset—such as the arrival of a
new brother or sister—he or she may temporarily
lose recently acquired skills, such as potty-training.
But a child who loses several skills progressively, especially if there is no obvious cause, should be evaluated
by a physician. A number of treatable brain disorders,
including a tumor or HIV infection, can cause this
developmental regression.

Tip 223:

If you have a family history of crib death, or an infant with "near-miss crib death," you can take some simple measures that will dramatically reduce the risk of a recurrence.

In babies in developed countries aged two months to six months, crib death is still the most common cause of death. The incidence has decreased dramatically since the public education campaigns of the early 1990s on the sleeping positions of babies. But even in countries that have seen a bigger drop in deaths than the United States, the crib death rate is rising slowly again as parents become complacent.

The following babies are especially at risk:

1. Premature and low-birth-weight babies.
2. Twins, triplets, etc. (multiple pregnancies)
3. Babies from a lower socioeconomic status.
4. Babies in households where anyone smokes, especially the mother. This risk increases with the number of cigarettes smoked. For every additional ten cigarettes per day, the risk of crib death increases threefold.

In order to dramatically reduce your baby's risk of crib death:

1. *Do not smoke* during pregnancy, or permit anyone to smoke in your household after the birth of your baby.

2. *Put your baby to sleep on his or her back.* If the baby has reflux (a spitting baby), tilt the baby on his or her left side to prevent fluid regurgitating into the lungs (aspiration). Once your baby is old enough to roll over, this is irrelevant.

3. *Do not overdress your baby* or use too much bedding, especially if the baby is already warm.

4. *If you think your baby is unwell, contact your doctor.*

5. *Breast-feed your baby* for at least 12 months if at all possible.

6. *Learn simple cardiopulmonary resuscitation (CPR) methods.*

6. *Never put a baby on a waterbed.*

Tip 224:

Infants and young children can easily swallow a wrong medicine or a dangerous household item (bleach, batteries, etc.). If a child does not talk, look for other signs in a case of poisoning with a toxic substance. If you are in doubt, call your Regional Poison Control Center for advice.

If your child has swallowed a potentially dangerous substance, it may be obvious—the child may tell you, or you may see the child with the container. But a child may also have swallowed a toxic substance unobserved. It may show itself in:

1. Sudden unusual behavior, dizziness, weakness, or illness

2. Abdominal pain, nausea, or vomiting
3. Blurred vision, a change in pupil size
4. Loss of bowel or bladder control

If you suspect that your child has swallowed a toxic substance, do the following:

1. **Stabilize your child.** Check their breathing and resuscitate if necessary (see Appendix A). Place them in the recovery position so that if they vomit, they will not choke. If the child is ill or not fully awake, call an ambulance (call 911 if available in your area).
2. **Identify the substance and amount swallowed.** Search carefully for any containers. If the substance was vitamin tablets with iron, for example, try to estimate the number missing from the container. If there are toxic chemicals on your child's skin, remove the contaminated clothes and wash the child with plain water. Get your child to an emergency room.
3. **If your child is stable, get advice on what to do.** Call your local poison control center (the number should be listed in your local phone directory under emergency numbers). Do not induce vomiting unless directed to do so.

You should never induce vomiting for:

1. Babies under six months
2. A child who is unconscious or who is having a seizure
3. A child who has already vomited profusely
4. A child who has swallowed a strong chemical (especially an alkali or acid), a petroleum product, or a solid object (glass, buttons, razors). Inducing

vomiting in these cases is dangerous, since it can cause complications in the esophagus (the tube leading from the mouth to the stomach) or lungs.

Do not wait for your child to become ill. Seek early advice. Delay can be fatal! Remember, the best way to save your child's life from poisoning is to not let him or her get near any toxic compounds. Store all your medicines and dangerous household items safely.

Tip 225:

Teenagers may abuse many substances (alcohol, tobacco, marijuana, solvents, Ecstasy, etc.) Inhaled solvents (glue, etc.) are especially dangerous and can cause brain, liver, and kidney damage and sudden death.

Substance abuse is more common in adolescent boys. Although tobacco is not a frequent cause of death among teenagers, alcohol is a major killer of both teenagers and adults. Solvent abuse may be harder to detect in your child, but excessive use of air fresheners may be a tipoff. Even a few "experiments" with solvents may result in long-term damage or death.

Watch out for personality change, major changes in mood or sleeping pattern, and appetite. Do not overreact. Try to be sure of your facts, and contact self-help groups for advice. If you are unsure whether your child is taking drugs, get professional help quickly. Do lead your children by positive example, and spend time with them so that they will trust you and know that you accept them.

Appendix A
Emergency Medical
Treatment

Often courses in the techniques to treat the following emergencies are available through the Red Cross, American Heart Association, or local hospitals. It is advisable to take these courses for in-depth training so you can be better prepared. Also, remember to ask someone to call for emergency help (911, etc.) while you are attempting to administer care.

•
Choking

The affected individual may have a sudden onset of coughing and redness or, more troubling, may be unable to cough or to speak and look blue in color. If it is a child with croup, suspected epiglotitis (see Tip 199), or asthma, do not undertake these procedures. You need to act rapidly before the person becomes limp and white.

Under the Age of One

Position: Place the infant facedown, with her head and neck below her trunk (e.g., on your knee). Support her neck and head with one hand.

Action: Using the heel of your other hand, give approximately five firm, quick blows between the shoulder blades. The object should shoot out.

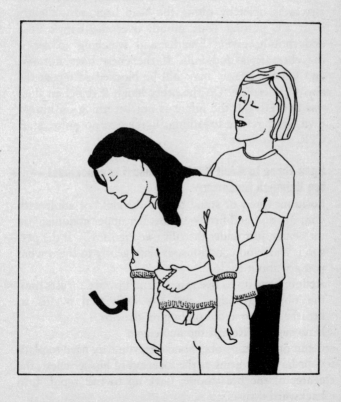

Figure 17. Heimlich Maneuver.

If no success: Turn her face-up on your lap or on a firm surface, and support her head and neck with one hand. Use two fingers of your other hand to thrust down five times in the center of her breastbone, directly between the nipples. Watch the mouth, and remove the object as soon as it appears.

If still no success: Call an ambulance (911 in most locations). If the infant is unconscious, check if the airway is open by tilting the head back very slightly if at all, putting your mouth over the baby's nose and mouth, giving breaths and watching to see if the chest rises and falls. If the chest does not rise and fall the airway may still be blocked so repeat the above procedure. On the other hand, if the chest does rise and fall but the infant is not breathing on his/her own, start rescue breathing. If there is no pulse, start CPR.

Ages Three to Adult (if the individual is conscious)— the Heimlich Maneuver

Position: Kneel or stand behind the child or adult with your arms joined firmly against her upper abdomen* in the center, just under the ribs (see Figure 17). If the person is alert and conscious, explain gently to them what you are about to do.

Action: Give up to five rapid, firm, upward thrusts until the object dislodges and the individual begins to breathe. Try to avoid pulling on the ribs.

If no success: Repeat the maneuver.

*In pregnant or obese persons, you may need to place your hands or arms at the location of his/her chest, the center of the breastbone. Give up to five rapid, firm backward thrusts.

Ages One to Three—(conscious or unconscious) or Ages Three to Adult (if unconscious):

1. Put the person on his or her back on a hard surface.
2. Kneel and straddle at the thighs facing the chest.
3. Place the heel of your hand just above the belly button.
4. Put your free hand on the positioned hand.
5. Provide five thrusts at a time in the midline, upward and inward.

Choking Prevention in Children

The best way to save a child from choking is to avoid it altogether. Children under three years of age are especially at risk, but the most difficult age group is from nine months to two years, when children are increasingly mobile and often put items in their mouth, but are not yet responsive to commands. Supervise your child well, and keep small items out of reach. Think carefully before giving your child certain foods.

Toys with Particular Risks

Balloons: Balloons are the most common cause of fatalities from choking. Always supervise children under the age of six when playing with balloons. Use Mylar, not latex balloons. Dispose of broken pieces of balloons immediately.

Small items: Avoid giving a child any item with small (under two inches) parts, especially coins, small balls, and toy food.

Small batteries: These are especially dangerous, as sometimes the acid can seriously damage the stomach lining.

Foods with Particular Risks

Nuts: This is the most commonly inhaled food. Do not give nuts to children under the age of five.

Hard candy: Do not give hard candy to children under the age of three.

Firm fruits or vegetables: Prepare carrots, grapes, apples, pears, and celery appropriately: Peel them, chop them finely, or cook them until soft.

Sausages: Give sausages to children over three if the skin is removed and they are well chopped.

Hot dogs: Cut hot dogs lengthwise, so that the bits are not in the shape of a coin.

•

Cardiopulmonary Resuscitation (CPR)

Any child or adult whose breathing or heartbeat stops will rapidly experience damage to their vital organs, especially the brain. Cardiopulmonary resuscitation (CPR) allows oxygen to reach the vital organs until expert help can be given in a hospital. This is a critical skill for you to learn. A written summary can give you only an outline; attending a CPR training course is the best way to learn.

CPR consists of a combination of:

1. Rescue breathing to get oxygen into the body
2. Chest compressions to distribute oxygenated blood throughout the body

The following steps are involved: A-A-B-C

Assess the situation and call for help
Airways: clear the airway
Breathing: rescue breathing
Circulation: chest compressions

Assess

Breathing: Look, listen, and feel for five seconds
Beating heart: Check for the pulse in the neck to feel if the heart is beating. In babies feel the upper inner arm with your fingertips.
Consciousness: Does the individual respond to you?
Other injuries: Are there other injuries? *Warning*—if you suspect a neck or spinal injury, do not move the person unless necessary!!
Call an ambulance (911 in most locations) if any of these apply:

- Not breathing
- Heart not beating
- Unconscious
- Other serious injury

Note: If an individual is experiencing any of the above, be aware that time is of the essence and you must start CPR immediately.

Airways

Position the victim on his or her back, ideally on a hard, flat surface. Log roll the victim to protect the neck and prevent possible additional injuries.
Extend his or her neck gently and lift the chin. This will open the airway. In an infant or child be careful not to bend the neck back, since this can block the airway.
Check to make sure that there are no objects in the mouth. Clear the mouth and throat.

Breathing

If an individual is not breathing, you must:

- (for baby) Put your mouth over the baby's mouth and nose.
- (for child or adult) Pinch the nose, and cover the mouth with your mouth.

Breathe into his or her mouth enough to inflate the chest. Breathe at a rate of 20 breaths per minute (once every three seconds); and 12 breaths per minute in adults.
Check that the chest moves. If not, consider the methods listed under Choking, to dislodge an object blocking the airway.

Circulation

If no heartbeat, act quickly:

For a baby

- Position your two fingers in the middle of the breastbone, level with the nipples.
- Press down about one inch, five times in three seconds.

For a child/adult

- Position the heel of your hand in the middle of the breastbone with your fingers pointing along the direction of the ribs. For adults, place the heel of one hand on top of the other. Be careful not to press on the ribs, only the breastbone.
- Press one and a half inches down. Follow the rescue breathing and chest compression rates listed below.

Combine rescue breathing and chest compressions according to the American Heart Association, as follows:

- Infants and children: Give five chest compressions and one rescue breath over a three-second period. Repeat the cycle.
- Adults: Give 15 chest compressions and two rescue breaths over a ten-second period. Repeat the cycle.
- Intermittently check the neck for a pulse, and if the pulse returns, then stop chest compressions but continue rescue breathing as long as the individual is not breathing on his/her own.

Do not give up until help arrives!!

Appendix B
Self-Examinations

Breast Exam

Perform an examination on your breasts at least once a month, preferably within the first week after your period. Regular examinations allow you to know what your breasts feel like normally so that you can readily detect any changes. Early detection and treatment of cancer increases the chance of a cure.

The following steps should be taken (see Figure 18):

1. Lie down flat on your back with a pillow under your right shoulder.
2. Place your right arm behind your head.
3. Press the pads of your three middle fingers firmly on your right breast. (A ridge in the lower curve of each breast is normal.)
4. Move your fingers around all parts of the breast, using a circular motion, an up-and-down motion,

or an in-and-out motion, around the circumference of a small circle. Use the same motions for the entire breast.

5. Put the pillow under your left shoulder, and follow the above steps to examine your left breast.

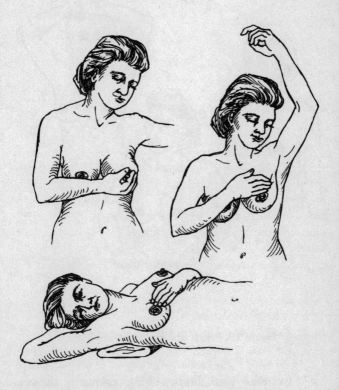

Figure 18. Breast Self-Exam, Palpation.

6. Stand in front of a mirror, and note any changes in the way your breasts look, such as dimpling of the skin, changes in the nipple, changes in the texture of the skin so that it resembles an orange peel, redness, or swelling (see Figure 19).

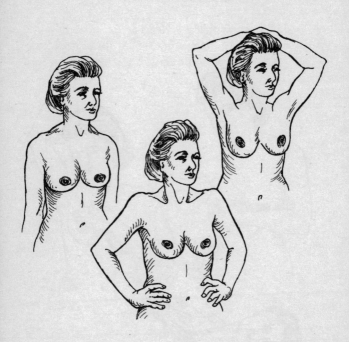

Figure 19. Breast Self-Exam, Observation.

7. Examine your breasts while taking a shower. Soapy hands over wet skin make it easy to check for lumps. Use similar technique as noted above.

8. If you find any changes, see your doctor right away.

•

Testicular Exam

Examine your testicles at least once a month (see Figure 20). You can do this in the shower in thirty seconds. Early detection and treatment of cancer can lead to a cure.

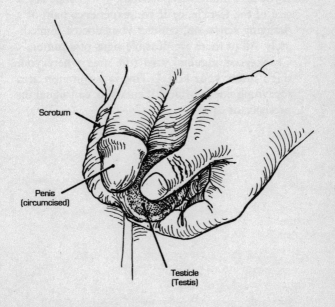

Scrotum

Penis
(circumcised)

Testicle
(Testis)

Figure 20. Testicular Self-Exam.

The following steps should be taken:

1. Place the scrotum between the thumb and the first three fingers.
2. Identify each testicle, which is smooth and round and feels like a hard-boiled egg. Each should move freely in your scrotal sac. You may feel a small crest of equal size and consistency in the back of both testicles, or on the edge of both testicles. This is a normal epididymis. Normal testicles should be of equal size without any differences. An abnormality in one testicle is rarely felt in the other.
3. If you find lumps, irregularities, or a change in the size of the testicle, or if you experience pain or a dragging sensation, contact your doctor immediately. All of these are possible signs of a tumor.
4. Check your inguinal area (the area where your thigh meets your body). This is a common area for lymph nodes, which, if enlarged, can signal the presence of cancer.

Index